The T*Ruth* About the Gift of Faith

by

Kaye Colello

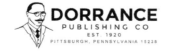
DORRANCE
PUBLISHING CO
EST. 1920
PITTSBURGH, PENNSYLVANIA 15238

Dorrance Publishing Co
585 Alpha Drive
Pittsburgh, PA 15238
Visit our website at *www.dorrancebookstore.com*

ISBN: 978-1-6495-7099-4
eISBN: 978-1-6495-7620-0

Dedicated to:

My loving and supportive husband and my two precious daughters, who taught me what true love really means. All of you are the co-authors of my life.

For more information on the
CARES FOUNDATION go to
www.caresfoundation.org

Chapters

Keep your thoughts positive because your thoughts become *YOUR WORDS*. Keep your words positive because your words become *YOUR BEHAVIOR*. Keep your behavior positive because your behavior becomes your *HABITS*. Keep your habits positive because your habits become *YOUR VALUES*. Keep your values positive because your values become *YOUR DESTINY*.

~Gandhi~

1

To Tell a Tale

Every person, at some point in their life, will have a story to tell of an event or of an experience endured that has, in some way, been life altering. That one event can render another human being that hears it speechless or fill them with awe. Not one living soul here on Earth will be exempt from a trial or lesson that is somehow inexplicably designed to teach acknowledgment, humbleness, and grace. Also, grow one in resilience and *thoughts*, as well as the character that inevitably alters a human being. All of us, in our lives, will experience one of these moments that are indelibly frozen in our memories of life. One never fully recovers from these events, be they so tragic or life-altering, that the spirit becomes wounded, nicked, and gouged from the pain inflicted upon it. The process of birth is once again placed upon the physical body, the pain wrought by the weight of millions of souls who have gone before each woman and man. One's conscious self, heart keening, and grievous sighing becomes a *memory* that leaves moist droplets of vaporous traces in the wind for those millions of people who will follow a painful path of *destiny.* They have traversed many roads only to experience suffering or happiness when they leave that mo-

ment behind. Eventually, the way gives rise to a thicket, where people strive to clear it so that the ones following will be safe, sound,
and mentally calm to usher in the future. Once a human emerges
through those laborious fog-filled tunnels of birth, we eventually
cross over to the other side of the thicket. As this occurs, the human
becomes passed into whom they will become and then comes to be
fortified in a new, organically industrialized kind of resilience that
speaks volumes to the power of the human spirit and one's *destiny*.

The two most powerful warriors are patience and time.

~Leo Tolstoy~

2

A Reckoning with TIME at High Noon

"They found a uterus." These four words divided our lives into two different planes of existence in this universe of ours. Like insects trapped in droplets of water, my husband and I felt as if we were restrained in a chamber of round walls from which we could not escape. Our minds confused, our souls attempted to bear the excruciating weight of human pain on us. It was as if our bodies and minds had gone into a form of suspended animation that we could not be resuscitated from. "They found a uterus;" words that would forever echo in the back of our minds, those words that initially evoked fear and grief at what they meant.

TIME is an elusive and infinite component in human existence that has been questioned since the beginning of ages. We, humans, have endeavored to slow it, categorize it, track it, chronicle it, write about it, and mathematically define it, yet we have never been able to harness nor travel through it. What exactly is *time*, and how does it define and mold one? I find myself often asking these questions but have yet to find the answer; however, there is one sure thing, and that is time is an elusive mist, fog, and smoke and mirrors construct. This false element in one's world controls humans day after day. It hones in on us, its victims, pausing silently for the individual's stopwatch to register high noon for a reckoning on life's gritty streets, but one never knows what the day will hold for them.

TIME weaves its spell silently in front of one's eyes, selling its wares to its unsuspecting buyers ever so quietly and cunningly. However, there are those naysayers that say that time is identifiable and then tick off in casual conversation. There are those ways it can be viewed and evaluated, such as the aging process itself, the trends made in fashion over the years, and even see and review the technological advances our world has made in science and medicine. But that is not the *time* I speak of.

TIME

I am speaking of *time* that is mentioned when one looks at a photo of their wedding day or prom night and says, "I remember that moment like it was yesterday," with a kind of melancholy reminiscence of adolescence lost and composure in their voice.

TIME

I refer to the kind of *time* that is spoken of on the everyday, familiar street corner in your neighborhood. The intersection where two old friends who may now be housewives or overworked businesswomen or men meet up and talk a good, well-deserved hour away before remembering they had other duties at home they must keep. The kind of *time* where a rapid glance at a watch elicits such statements as, "Oh my, look at the *time*! I have to get going now." Then they exchange their loving yet solemn goodbyes with the desire to recollect those youthful days when immortality was theirs for the taking.

TIME

I am speaking of that elusive *time* that we all experience when we finally realize our mortality in life as we watch our children ride off on two-wheel bicycles, graduate, or get married. We ask ourselves silently, "Where did all the time go? It has just slipped away from me, and I didn't even recognize it; life goes by so fast...how I wish I could do this again," as a mixed bag of raw and unedited emotions churn in one's bowels and course through our minds. Standing in front of a mirror can also be painful, as the gravity of time has plans to pull us down in the physical state of aging, face sagging, and our youth stripped away. Days end our concept of *time* by pulling us beneath the earth where one can rest for eons.

THAT TIME

That time is invisible, only it is not, and it performs its magical duties in real time as a human weaver of traditions and morals that becomes the foundation of cultural and societal rules that we must learn to abide by here in this world. *That time.* That time that makes us say and do odd things during times of stress because of those boundaries and rigid rules one has grown up with. *That time.* That *time* that familiarized the generic neighborhood corner conversations that are held in every nook and cranny of the world. *This time,* the one that makes one's memories fade yet reminds us how short life really is and how sweetly precious and most pure moments are. *That time.*

Although mostly invisible to the naked eye, the only tangible evidence of time's presence in personal development are the subtle or sometimes sharp lines of change that affect human lives. Once we can look back in hindsight with strength, it allows us to see the changes *time* has sold us in precise, three-dimensional forms. This glance over the shoulder enables you to bring mindfulness, patience, and yearning to mind for a broader realization as it replays life's moments with clarity behind one's strength. It has always followed one's path within the deepest recesses of the mind, heightening the senses, allowing you to reach out and touch and feel your testimony, such as pain or happiness of the event. It recalls events and milestones, both high and low, that have shaped who we have become. The analysis of the dismembered self and dysfunctional outcomes of our missteps comes from all angles, and by doing this, one remembers the joy and pain in one's life, putting our immediate moment back in place. Time is the only way *time* can be measured, and at the moment of realization, we feel change has been a positive or negative one. A human has to eventually learn, with patience, to accept time's gift and make the best of it, leaving your shadow to fall behind you and face upturned to the sun.

I learned, and because of this, my glance back to the past events and silhouettes leading to the Gift of Faith are now focused on the clarity that can be humanly distinguished by having 20/20 vision. There isn't a day that goes by that I don't reflect on my life before and after Faith, the happiness I have found and how I came to rest where I am today.

Once upon a time, I was adrift on the sea of life, floating through it with my eyes wide shut, riding the swells of life that brought me one bump at a time, hoping, as I crested over a wave, that whatever rested on the other side would be manageable. Nevertheless, *time* changed that existence for me, sneaking in with a willowy and ethereal hand. It caressed my face like a well-seasoned lover. It then lulled me and whispered sweet nothings in my ear to confuse me, just as the rhythmic lapping of the ocean will do on the hull of a dinghy cast adrift on an uncertain sea. *Time* became the ancient navigator in my life, attracting its power from all the natural elements of the east, west, north, and south, and compiling them into one microcosmic juncture that would erupt into the macrocosm of change. Time blew salt-laden winds of definitive change into my eyes, blinding me from the person I was before. Then, with the gritty substance embedded, my vision was blurred in liminal space, taking time itself to encourage me to refocus my sights on what it had provided to my first class, teaching about the oceanic garden of life to the oceanic qualities of my womb.

Then, to the hour, to the minute, to the second, with precise timing, my life's clock ticked up that monumental moment of change, and with a crescendo, I became poised briefly for a moment on the wind and then traversed beyond, spiraling downward and crestfallen as my new reality took a hold of me. By mere seconds, two of them to be exact, side by side on a clock face, time became the catalyst that would forever change my life. Strength, a powerful warrior, formally acquainted itself with patience to show me what my future would hold in its hands.

Principals are profound fundamental truths… lightly interwoven threads running with exactness, consistency, beauty, and strength through the fabric of life.

~Steven Covey~

3

The Fabric of Many Colors

I purchased my first home fifteen years after mama passed away. It was a luxurious and fully renovated condominium that boasted every modern amenity available in an old Victorian mansion built for a ship's captain. This ancient boat captain's house overlooked the Quinnipiac River in New Haven, Connecticut. There was a sense of pride in myself for having purchased my first home with good old-fashioned arduous work as an operations manager for a Fortune 500 company in the home improvement industry. I was on top of my game in life, driving a fancy new car and the proud owner of a stylish home. The dutiful working daughter had acquired her version of the American dream. There were many times I thought my mother would be proud of me and how I wished she were still alive to see my accomplishments.

It was in that same time frame of my life that I encountered my future husband, Joey, a man of Italian descent whose stiff New England traditions were far different from my relaxed, West Coast upbringing. He captivated me with his thick eastern accent and old-fashioned standards, and I found his way curiously mesmerizing. It were those simple things that made me interested in a complicated way of life that was so different from my own.

Joey was the ideal model of the Italian American male; he was impeccably dressed, neatly shaved, and hair in place. Although I was delighted when he asked me out the first night we met, I distinctly remember eyeing his hair and wondering how much hairspray and gel he must go through in a year. Me? I wore none. Him? At least a can and a half. Regardless, I accepted the date, hair, and all, and with that, our relationship began to weave itself into a fabric of many colors.

Over time, he and I developed a fun-loving yet profoundly caring relationship where we soon came to recognize we wanted it to last. Proposals of marriage and children dotted our discussions, but our cultural distinctions made taking the final step slippery. However, the nature of life eventually became a deep, fundamental, and silent agreement that developed. This demonstrated our attempts to try and understand each other for what we stood for, not imagining in our youth whom we would marry. Many initiated symposia took place between us as we struggled with learning about each other's distinctions, family, and arguing about various lifestyles. We marveled at our parallels and argued over differences. Joey and I came from broken homes, yet he had the experience of having a father in the house growing up, until the divorce happened to him, whereas I did not have any experience at all.

Joey would heartily reminisce about his life as a young boy, periodically rambling on for hours with stories and anecdotes of the life he cherished, where my storied narratives of happy times were sparingly infrequent if not rarely retold to him. He was born at Yale-New Haven Hospital, raised in Hamden, Connecticut, and spiritually nurtured as a Catholic amidst family and friends. Some of whom were first-generation Italians. He would describe in

great detail his boyhood growing up in an Italian American neighborhood where family ties were thick, the bonds of friendship
steady, neither of which extended far beyond their area. One of
my favorite family ramblings was Joey's descriptions of Sunday
dinners at his grandparent's home, which never failed to make
me hungry. The details of his Nona's pot of sauce, simmering on
the stove with meatballs sizzling in a pan, were enough to make
a girl want that type of familial setting for her own. The loaves of
warm Italian bread and those excellent Italian pastries, enough to
feed an army, made me wonder what his Nona's house must have
smelled like to him as a child. How beautiful life must have been
for him growing up and how nice to be able to possess, or at least
paint, colorful threads with so many beautifully decorated memories of a childhood surrounded with family and bonded by the
warmth of food.

Joey, the oldest of three sons, was always at his father's side
when the opportunity presented itself. He put his father on a
pedestal, and one of his fondest memories as a little boy was the
smell of wood chips on his father's clothing when he came home
from work. His father was a carpenter by trade and was dusted in
those intoxicatingly earthy smells. Joey also looked forward to snug-
gling up to his dad while in front of the television. There they would
wait for supper by his mother. Joey's mother always worked hard
at keeping her family happy by maintaining a clean home and de-
licious meals on the table. Joey loved his mother deeply for all her
efforts and would often marvel at how she managed to keep the
house going with so many men in her care. If there was one thing I
knew for sure, it was that he loved and cherished the memories of
that time in his life, always bringing up her stained-glass cookies.
As Joey had aged and life manifested itself, he missed the joy of
childhood more and more. His heart desperate because his family

structure was dramatically altered in his nineteenth year by a divorce that divided and changed the family dynamics forever.

On the other hand, my naivety stood out in stark contrast to Joey's. Most of my memories were fraught with despair and fear that I cared not to relive very often. When I did, it left me feeling vulnerable and unable to protect myself from the world, and the stinging questions that may arise might ask me of my upbringing.

Me? I was born in Merced, California, at Mercy Hospital, amongst cow farming towns nestled amongst fruit orchards. I, too, was nurtured in the Catholic faith. My family consisted of a loosely strung together poor lot of kids who did not match in father or color, and who had no father or male figure in the home. We were the amalgamation of a rainbow. I was the youngest of five siblings, with a total of three different fathers between us. The oldest two siblings shared a father, as did the next two, and then there was me with no siblings in common. My sibling set spread out over a considerable period of time, the oldest, about sixteen years old when I was born, and the youngest being me. We had nothing but each other, and even that was strained, and when our mother fell ill with heart trouble, it was that time our lives fell into dire straits. The two oldest siblings went off to live with their father while the remaining three of us spent two years in different foster homes due to our mother's long-term recovery from heart surgery at Palo Alto by a doctor named Shumway. He did a phenomenal job because, after that, she had a long recovery. Once she returned home, she attempted to restore normalcy for the four of us while the oldest two siblings never returned home.

Mama scraped for every morsel of food that went on the table and every item of clothing she could get her hands on. She saved every penny she could and, by my sixth birthday, had managed to save up five hundred dollars to move us away from specific individuals that circulated a letter accentuating her undesirability in the workforce due to her "promiscuity" resulting in her "mulatto" children. With that five hundred dollars, Mama eventually relocated us to San Diego, a place she dreamed of living in and giving her children a better and more diverse way of life. After some searching, we eventually found affordable, government-subsidized apartments in southeast San Diego, and it was there, in Bay Vista Methodist Heights, that we settled in for the long haul of life on our own.

Mama struggled to keep us afloat, working until she could no longer do it. Her illness eventually made her weak and unable to continue in the workforce.

Stories about me crying in my crib, wanting to be held, abounded, but she wouldn't allow herself to speak about such a painful part of her life. More stories were told about the family, such as she would be hemorrhaging blood from her lungs and was incapable of caring for us. My two big sisters cared for me while Mama found out what her illness was. It was then she had to turn to state aid to feed us as we watched her health slowly deteriorate over time. Eventually, both sisters had grown old enough to leave home and start their own families. The oldest of the three of us was stationed in the Philippines with her husband who was a member of the United States Air Force. The second sister relocated to Tucson, Arizona, with her husband, who was also a member of the Air Force. She never moved out of our home until the age of twenty-seven, feeling the need to care for Mama and me. Once she did leave, I was the last sibling at home and, therefore, left alone with Mama to care for her and perform all the tasks that she could no longer do, which was almost everything. The family I was accustomed to was gone, whittled away by *time* to just the two of us, Mama and me.

I shopped for groceries, went to the laundromat, and escorted Mama to her doctor's appointments all the while attempting to juggle high school, a social life, and survive being a teenager. My growth as a teenager was interrupted as I was forced into adulthood prematurely. In our family setting, there were no longer family meals or get-togethers and no savory smells emitting from our kitchen. Instead, I cooked my own TV dinners or bowls of instant ramen noodles. Sustenance was doled out carefully in our house, and I had to ask for every morsel I wanted because Mama and I were on a tight state budget and couldn't afford to be snacking whenever the urge struck us. For our family, the kitchen was not central to the heartbeat of our home, rather the living room was. Keeping a roof over our heads seemed to be the harsh and stark reality that outweighed that lovely kitchen idea.

There it was, in all its nakedness, childhood wasn't terribly joyful for me. I was always fraught with fears far beyond those that a young child should ever have to face. My worries centered on where our next meal would come from and what would become of me should Mama die. She must have known I was worried because her favorite saying was, "Whatever you do in life, I will always be proud of you, but make sure whatever it is that you do, be the best at it." Mama also used to say, to be able to get through life's adversities, one must do so with their heads held high and faces turned up to the sky while your shadow falls behind you. "Remember," she would say, "the Lord has plans to prosper you and not to harm you." I tried my best to follow her words of wisdom, but there were many nights I cried myself to sleep, demanding to know why this fate was prescribed to me, and how was it fair? All around me I saw people my age with mothers and fathers, beautiful homes to live in, and a way of life so foreign to me, I wondered what it would be like to live like them, to be like them. My life was different from my peers; my life seemed destined to serve the role of a caregiver. However, others my age seemed blessed enough to be able to enjoy their youthfulness with carefree thoughts and actions that had no barriers, no predicaments, and no dangerous illnesses to threaten their safety net.

As I grew older, there were many occasions where Mama would call me to her bedside and tell me not to fear and relate to me how she had gone to church to pray before her heart surgery. She prayed to God that she would live to see her youngest child, me, graduate from high school. On one occasion, she told me that she had been talking with a priest in the hospital before she came home from her surgery and told him of her prayer. His response to her was, "Well, you have already asked the Lord for that blessing, and God answers prayers, so now it is time to ask Him for something else." She loved retelling that story to me, and she must have loved how it made me smile; only there was *fear* hiding inside me and the smiles, fake. As I became older, the smile I could manage became smaller and smaller. I began to fear my growth into adulthood, knowing that if the Lord did answer prayers, my mama's *time* on earth was rapidly coming to a close. And then it happened.

Mama had gone away once again to the hospital, and I was left all alone to fend for myself in the house after school let out. Every other day, on the way home from school, I would make the drive to the hospital to see her and would have to park in the lot at the bottom of a steep hill because there were never any parking spots in the lot at the top. My memory painfully and profoundly reminds me of how I hated that long walk up the hill from the second parking lot to the first one in the sweltering San Diego heat, wishing I didn't have to come. The only thing I looked forward to was the automatic doors at the entrance to the hospital. The doors seemed as if they were waiting to ominously greet me when they gaped apart, spilling out a swoosh of cool hospital air as I approached and they opened. Strangely and uncomfortably, it felt like those doors had been expecting me all day long, waiting patiently for me to enter into their house of ills. It was there, in that hospital, nothing more than a giant box where both ill and deceased people lay. My mother lay in her sickbed, biding her time to come to an end, and I despised every moment of the idea of it. I despised it because, at that moment in time, the hospital did not represent healing to me but rather the slow and imminent death of someone I loved more than life itself. It didn't represent hope for the future, but rather it placed me in a holding pattern where I circled death like vultures over a dying creature. And so there, at the hospital, I hovered, scared out of my wits, waiting for the landing strip to become the end of the trip of profound sadness. I was circling the airport of doom, waiting to crash and land in the same spot where those who lost loved ones before me were waiting with sunken eyes and hollowed out hearts for a time to make them whole again.

I, the dutiful daughter, would enter those doors and make my way, every other day, carefully to the elevators, my head down watching where each step was placed so that I could pick my way around the green tiles that contained spirits being escorted to and from their old to new homes by heavenly messengers. I would cover my nose and mouth with my hand and take small and shallow breaths in the grand hallway of the hospital to ensure I did not breathe too hard. Fear ruled my every move, and I didn't want to inhale the essence of those departing on their airline. I was strangely afraid that death would follow me to her room. I imagined the unknowing pawn could bring an end to the door of an unwitting family who was spending joyful last minutes with their loved one. I did not want to bring death to the door of my mother; I wanted her room hidden from the one ethereal entity responsible for escorting those dearly departed to another realm.

Once on my mother's floor, I would wind my way through the corridors to her room where the odors of sickness and faded life laced its fingers in my nose and through my brain. My mother would greet me with a weak hello, and I greeted her with a kiss. There we would sit, her telling me what I needed to do at home and me, the obedient daughter, would sit quietly, taking her orders down on paper. The usual conversations would always take place such as what I did at school that day or what I was planning on eating for supper, but nothing of earth-shattering proportions were ever really discussed in that room. Perhaps I avoided anything too deep, too precarious, or too fragile to carry my utterances through the air around me in conversation, and so, instead, I danced a light number with my mother so she could not see my grief. I could flit from one note to the other without getting bogged down under the heaviness of my heart. After an hour or so, she would send me on my way, knowing I needed to get home, and therefore, she urged me to call her when I did reach home so that she wouldn't worry. That was our special routine that did not last very long.

Eventually, she couldn't speak anymore, and so, she resorted to writing me notes on scraps of paper, telling me that everyone has to die. Another note would ask what I had to eat for supper. Those notes were more than I could stomach, but somehow, I couldn't part with them; they contained her mana, her energy, her spirit, her endurance that was kept alive in each stroke of the pencil on paper. She struggled to write, and watching this, I knew I could not, would not, ever part with them. To me, those papers were her essence that I would always be able to touch and feel no matter how far away from me she would travel in this universe of ours. Once she passed beyond my ability to see her anymore physically, I would be intertwined in a waiting game with time to see her again.

That fateful day of dark and frozen memory still haunts me today. The phone began to ring mid-morning and then continued all afternoon with strange callers asking who my mother's next of kin was. It never dawned on me what they were calling for until my sister Bernadette called from Tucson several hours later. She broke the news to me; Mama had passed away the night before, at 3:30 in the morning. There I sat, my mouth agape and tears streaming down my face. I was writhing on the floor screaming for my mother while clinging to the black bean bag only to realize she passed on at the same time she appeared to me in a dream. The night before I had dreamed of her, and at that exact *time* I shot straight up in bed drenched in a cold sweat. I stared at the clock; it was 3:30 a.m., and I was scared, scared because my mother had spoken to me with her solid chocolate eyes and face spinning and spinning, and all the while, her voice called my name. When the spinning stopped, she was very close to me, and she begged me to take her off of her breathing machine. Now she was gone, and it dawned on me that Mama got *her* prayers answered because she had lived long enough to see me graduate from high school. However, my world was wholly and utterly shattered into a million shards of glass so tiny that I could never put them back together again. My heart had finally been torn to shreds, my spirit hollowed out like a ripe melon in the summer, and my mind could take no more. Somehow, I would have to reconcile all of this pain to find some peace in her death, but it would have to wait until *time* had passed me by. After all, they do say that *time* heals all wounds, don't they? But who are *they* and what do *they* know about time? *That time*. The quiet time that passes one by with the slightest of breezes while they're dozing on an insignificant dinghy on the most unpredictable day within the sea of life that encompasses the world.

With the help of my two sisters and friends, I managed to survive Mama's passing, but I struggled alone to learn how to grow into a full-fledged adult. Although I had been forced into being a grown-up when it came to household responsibilities and the caring of my mother, I was still a child at heart. The actualization that I was alone in the world without the comfort of a mother's love frightened me terribly and scarred me horribly. At least when Mama was there, she guided me in all aspects of growth. But now, suddenly, in the blink of an eye, *time* had ripped a portion out of the floorboard of my spirit. The rip in my spirit caused me to spring a leak. The vital force which drove me daily to forge ahead seemed to have emptied from the cut, right out of me into a puddle on the bottom of the sea. The loss was so massive for me to try and overcome that it made me a victim of the sea. I began to sink into the vast ocean of grief that stared blankly back at me. I was in the doldrums. I peered over the edge of the boat I was riding on to get through this moment and stared into the abyss of life, eyes wide open and wild with fear as there was no movement. The restrictions of time had left me motionless in spirit as I sat in the doldrums, a place where east meets west, and a sort of silence and minimal movement transpires. I was stuck between life and death and wished to move on where the sea could carry my soul. The ravages of time had at first left me tossed about in the waves of existence with nowhere to go. So I would turn to those messages she had scribbled on to paper for me, on those scraps of paper I had provided for her and her voice when she couldn't speak anymore. They were the comfort pills that I could hold onto and get high on until I was ready to sail on. They held her essence, her handwriting, her power at the end of her life. In turn, I resurrected her memory from them, hopelessly searching for that mundane continuity of conversation that happened at that period in time. *Time* was what I so dreaded, all the while holding the notes, awash in guilt in my heart, and asking for forgiveness for my sins by hating the visits to the hospital. I still have those notes tucked away in a shoebox today, and every once in a while, I glance at the contents that are too powerful to throw away. The words and memories bring me to tears, but the contents of that shoebox are my most cherished possession.

Today, I wonder about young people who use texting and computers to communicate. What will become of the intimacy of having a loved one's handwriting to be able to trace your finger on and view something they penned with their hand once they are gone if we do not physically write anymore. My mother's penmanship is a treasure that is irreplaceable and far more valuable to me than any email she could have ever typed to me at the end of her life. When I hold her notes, it is like I can hold her once again in the palm of my hand.

Over time I became embattled and bitter by my life's dice throw and trying to make my way through each situation I encountered as a motherless daughter became increasingly frustrating. So, listening to Joey's anthology of childhood tales didn't make me feel better about my lot in life. I often envied him, jealous that I didn't have a family connection of that magnitude growing up. For years, I was so wrapped up in my self-pity and jealousy that I failed to see the blessing God had bestowed on Mama by answering *her* prayers.

Thinking back, the symbolism of the black bean bag became the color of my heart.

Joey and I were beginning a new chapter in life where our stories would bind together, and our relationship would become the selvage edge of a fabric that would weave a family history. It was then the fabric I had woven for years before I met him was buried deep in the pit of my stomach. For he and I, the fabric consisted of two separate pasts. In a few short years, we would be woven together more tightly than we could have ever imagined. Perhaps the scripture in the Bible that Mama had spoken about was true; maybe God *did* have plans for me.

No one besides Allah can rescue a soul from hardship

~Qur'an 53:58~

4

Dream a lot of Dreams of Me

Dreams are funny little snippets in our lives, all jumbled up in our sleep, creating a patchwork of dreamscapes and moments that are haphazardly stitched together. It leaves no sense of time or order. When particular swatches of time in life are trapped in this way, it can elicit feelings that paint a canvas of questions for dreams far too sweeping to be answered; however, it leaves one obvious question, "What was that dream all about?" Then there are those dreams rarely as brilliant as a bell's peal; those dreams that are interpreted as succinctly as the tribal storyteller recounts history around a crackling fire on a dark, steamy night. Those dreams are so powerful in imagery and messages that no matter how many years ago the reel to reel was left to flap noisily around the unattended projector of the mind's eye, the picture remains as vividly clear as if you watched the plot of your own story unfold in a movie. I was scared, but I knew God would rescue my soul. When? I did not know if it were God that would *really* RESCUE it. Would it be me, an unrecognized human being, or a turn for the better in my soul? I wasn't sure if anything had ever been clear cut for me.

I wasn't much of a dreamer, in my sleep, that is, but I had dreams and aspirations in life that I wanted to fulfill. So, after long discussions over what to do as far as a future with Joey was concerned, a decision was finally reached that had me leaving my job, getting married, and starting a family. Although I agreed to that scenario, there was still great hesitance on my part. Half of me was excited that a new chapter in my life was beginning, but the other half of me found it hard to leave the life experience I had finally created for myself.

I had floated about on a vast sea in that little dinghy of mine for many years, and often pictured myself as Hemingway's character from *The Old Man and the Sea*, adrift in the ocean with a big fish lashed to the side of my rickety boat, which was my life. With oar raised, I had pounded off each predator that took turns eating away at what I had fought and labored to gain in my life for years. By the time I was a young adult, I felt there were hardly any bits or pieces left on my fish (life). Therefore, traversing puddles, ponds, and lakes in my journey here on earth, I wasn't so sure I was ready to surrender those small victories to the whims of someone else's dreams and goals, especially when they weren't in alignment with mine.

Joey owned a three-family home that was a rundown, aging ark of a structure that in my opinion was more suitable for a hungry fire than a family. The house was big and gangly in form and stood amongst others of its kind, all of which were decrepit and in need of extensive repairs. It smelled of mothballs and liniment oil, most assuredly the odors of former residents both living and long since passed away that still lingered. Envisioning living alongside those ghosts of Hamden's past didn't suit me well; the thought was enough to give me cold feet and a nagging feeling in the deep recesses of my mind that there would be something of the otherworld sort of watching me sleep.

As the move-in date approached, the decision I had initially made became a certainty I could no longer reconcile in my mind. Looking to place blame for my decisions, I grew increasingly agitated with Joey and let my frustrations fly with no restraint or regard for his feelings. On more than one occasion, in a fury, I let loose the fact that I could not believe I had agreed to the arrangement. I did not care if I wounded him with the barbed spears I hurled through the air in the form of words and with tantrum-throwing, yet I still pitifully dragged my feet towards my new life, groaning and complaining all the way. After two weeks of throwing those fits and trying to come to some peace and acceptance with the changes that were happening in my life, I found that I was still depressed. Joey tried his best to be supportive of me, but there was nothing anyone could have done to have brought me out of the funk I was living in. I was out of sorts, out of a job, and scared that I might have, once again, made a wrong decision in my life.

One night in my new (old) home, I laid in bed and cried while Joey slept, bewildered at how drastically my life had changed and how I had allowed it to happen. I hated the new digs and wanted the comforts of my old home back again. Here in the strange outpost of the unknown, one could hear every footstep taken and conversations held by the other two families living above us, limiting any privacy to be had. I may have been accustomed to living in my old house, and this way of life exposed me once again to the apartment-style living I remembered and despised as a child. I felt that frightened little girl's fears and worries that I had fought so hard to cut out of my life wash over me while I drifted off into a fitful and tumultuous sleep.

"*How did I get here?*" I asked myself in a strained whisper of thought while standing in the backyard of the three-family home. "*Why am I standing so still? Why can't I move?*" Somehow, I had managed to get myself out of the rear of the house and into the backyard. There I stood, stiff as a zombie staring off into space. The odd thing about this whole situation I found myself in was that I had just gone to bed for the evening, meaning that it was dark outside when I retired, but now it was broad daylight, perhaps even high noon, because the sun was directly overhead, hanging high like an overripe pumpkin in the sky. With the sun beating down on my head, it made the whole scenario strangely bizarre. TIME had been skewed in some way here in the backyard of **NEVER-land,** and I asked myself, *"Am I dreaming?"* Somewhere faintly in the distance, I could hear the strained yet familiar lyrics of "Dream a Little Dream of Me," drifting through the air. The words crackled and skipped as they played out on an anonymous neighbor's record that drifted to my ears on the breeze.

There, appearing on the right side in my peripheral vision, I made out the figure of a being that I knew was not there a moment ago. There was also something deep inside me that warned me not to look in that direction because my human self would not be able to withstand the magnitude of the power He possessed. Somehow, there was an unsaid understanding that glancing over and laying eyes on whomever or whatever was standing there beside me would have stopped my heart, DEAD…in midbeat. He said, "You cannot see my face, for no man can see my face and live." Then, standing rigidly, I felt the hair on the back of my neck prickle as the figure leaned in towards me. I trembled and lowered my eyes to the ground, not knowing what to expect, yet somehow, I was not frightened. Cupping hands to my head, the figure blew breath gently into my ear; the gentle gust was His voice, a language which was articulated to me like melodic sounds of otherworldly chimes blowing in the breezes of heaven itself. This powerful gesture seized me in its grip and dropped me to my knees instantaneously. Like a stone that has been hurled into the depths of the sea, I didn't gracefully fall to my knees; instead, I sank, hitting the pavement as if my legs were knocked out from under me. He had spoken, and the message commanded me to fall on bended knee. As these events transpired, *time* virtually stood still in the dreamscape. Everything slowed and became magnified so that the ungrateful wretch that had been called upon could process the message. Experiencing the dream made me think of in real-time a heavenly version of *The Dummies Handbook for Callings*, with the byline blaring, "Expressly written for WRETCHES" becoming indelibly inked in my mind.

Imagine if you would have a dream shown to you in freeze-frame, with every item you see and experience becoming magnified so that every detail created could be seen with clarity. This is how I saw everything for the next few minutes of my dream. I could hear my heart roughly drumming in my ears, beating rhythmically to the wonders of life and Mother Earth. All vibrations of the world coursed through my body. I looked into the sky as I began to be cleansed with a heightened sense of awareness of just how magnificently created every single object, creature, and human existed. We were the only ones on the face of this earth that might be able to work compassionately with each other at this point in the dream. It was then I realized I wasn't on the ground but in the sky, floating. Blades of grass were brought to eye level so that I could see each crystalline drop of dew. The flight of the hummingbird was slowed down so that each beat of its tiny wings matched the thump, thump, thumping of my heart. I could count each flap of them with ease, and every detail of its beautiful iridescent feathers could be scrutinized. As each wondrous vision was shown to me, I realized how precisely unique and put together everyone and every living thing are. Then, in my mind, the breath translated into a message for me, and that message was, "I have *something* I want you to do, and *every-*

thing will *be okay.*" The great creator had cured my soul. He actually came to save me. Quick as He appeared, He was gone, and I felt a sudden sadness come over me that I was alone again. However, I knew that I must tell others on my block about the joyful message since I was back on earth. So, I began a frantic rush from door to door in my neighborhood gathering neighbors together to tell them what had just happened. Some joined me in the street where we gathered in a circle on bended knee. Turning our faces skyward, we reached out our arms in praise of the wonder and benevolent gift of faith. FADE TO BLACK, and then I slept soundly and quietly for the rest of the night.

The next morning, I awoke with the dream burning in my mind just as fresh as if it had taken place in real-time. Having experienced something beyond my realm of understanding and out of reach of what my imagination could have ever conceived on its own, the mere thought of the dream would reduce me to tears. I would sit and try to make sense of something that I couldn't make any sense of, and as I would spread the facts out in my brain like a deck of cards, I could see that there was no logic to the dream because the cards kept shuffling in my mind as if I were in a card game; therefore, at that time of looking for an answer, I could not find it. The hand I held was a bad deal, leaving me to play with the hand I was dealt. There was no rhyme or reason. It simply wouldn't make any sense to a reasonable and sound-minded individual, and the events of this dream weren't making any sense to me. Yet, this dream was very real, and I could replay it over and over again as if I had just dreamed it mere seconds ago. It became a real sporting event, sort of like a football outing with me being the sole fan at my very own tailgate party. I would sit and recall the dream blow by blow that made it like it was a real-life football event being played back on instant replay with the voice on mic blaring out the plays that took place in the dream on that fateful field of AstroTurf in my mind. Each move would be carefully noted and critiqued as I played them out in my brain. Curiously, each vibrant color was real and undisturbed. This dream was different, and I knew it. That was what made it so frightening in a supernatural yet genuine sense.

I knew I needed to write down the dream, knowing I had just experienced something unique. I wanted to ensure the memory had been recorded on paper so that one day I would be able to share this dream with others. TIME has a distinct and methodical way of making details fade, so I scribbled them down and put the paper in an envelope inside of our safe. As the days passed by, I came up with many questions in mind while mulling over this powerful dream. Questions like, *Would this be a turning point in my life that hadn't been revealed to me yet? Was I going to be blessed with any more dreams such as this?* I hoped so, but what was I supposed to wait for?

For two weeks I kept the dream a secret from Joey and everyone else I knew, afraid that he and the others would scoff at me in disbelief. Let's face the facts; this wasn't the kind of everyday dream a friend or family member relates to you. Especially seeing how the person recounting it insists that the dream was more than a dream that had happened, sort of, in a dream state kind of way, yet it was real. I could envision people talking behind my back saying how strange I was and how I needed to rest to clear my mind of that sort of nonsense. So, to avoid the embarrassment of any kind, I ran the events of the dream over in my head once again, then tucked it away deep in the pit of my stomach, convincing myself that I was an outlet of some sort to make me feel better again. There was a moment I felt the urge to be of service to others, and in my mind, I thought I might be needed at every food pantry and do-good organization in town. Finally, I had it figured out; I was supposed to volunteer my time at a local soup kitchen down at one of the churches in the neighborhood. That's what I was called upon to do, of course! How could I have possibly missed that one? After all, isn't that what every do-gooder such as myself with a mission to fulfill does? Spend a short time volunteering, ladle some food out, and make yourself feel better by talking about it to some friends. Then, make yourself feel even better than before because you told so many people what you did to help those in need, thus elevating yourself even higher on the "holier than thou" food chain, *I'm going to heaven before you because of my good work at the soup kitchen.* Yeah, I thought, that's what I'll do. Brownie points never hurt anyone, especially *getting into heaven* brownie points.

Well, guess what happened. I never volunteered at the soup kitchen. Not that soup kitchen anyway, and for the record, I'm not being cynical about service to others; we humans do give out of the goodness of our hearts, but we sometimes serve for other strange and convoluted reasons, like bragging rights. I didn't want that to be why I would volunteer and worried that there, tucked away somewhere deep down inside my soul, that very reason might be lurking. I imagined it to be floating around in my subconscious, clamoring to broadcast the good deed I thought I was about to perform. If I did do that, it would validate me as a true believer in a higher authority than my peers and mark me with the highly coveted badge of "SERVICE TO OTHERS." I didn't like that much, so there were moments that my cynicism for this thought rose up like vomit in my throat, turning me away from making any call to volunteer my time. Anyway, I was just too caught up in second-guessing myself. Maybe I was just too lazy, or perhaps I just plain out knew deep down inside that the soup kitchen gig was really **NOT** what I was supposed to do. Why? Because it **NEVER** manifested itself in my life at that particular time. Something else eventually did. However, for whatever reason, time wasn't ready to reveal the task; I was going to have to wait a little while longer.

Two weeks after having the dream, I discovered I was pregnant. For as long as I could remember, I had never wanted children and had managed to make it to my thirty-third year of life without any, and quite frankly, I liked it like that. As I viewed it, children represented a huge change in life and nothing more. In my eyes, the only purpose they served was to throw a wrench into your plans, which ultimately changed everything in your life for worse. Because of the mindset, and because of my own childhood, thoughts of children turned me away. I implemented and followed a strict personal policy that systematically removed friends from my friendship as they married and had children. Those friends inevitably became boring people who did nothing but recite every minute the cute detail they thought their child had done or said, "Billy took his first steps today; Robin turned five months old today." You see it on Instagram and Facebook, sending out a subliminal message, *Don't forget to like my picture.* Well, those stories did nothing for me, but I donned my poker face, then my surprised face, and then I opened up my can of laughter, smiles and fake concern to get myself together so as not to hurt their feelings. All my laughter and pleasantries about an incident made me a liar. I was not interested at all in what their children were up to, and to top it off, they seemed to never be free of those kids when we got together to catch up just like old times of our comings and goings. Their kids were like weights, and they, my friends, had human chattel attached to them. I would manage to sit and commiserate for a time, but my relationship with an old friend grew further and further apart because half of her attention was directed towards her little one. When one does not want children, then the feeling of separating from friendship becomes easier to understand.

Eventually, I became strained, due to the child that was always vying for my girlfriend's attention. Then, when the friend noticed how time had gotten away from her and she had to run off to fix dinner for her husband, I could swear I would catch that wistful longing for the past in her eyes. She was no longer the most vibrant friend I once knew, but instead, she was unusually haggard and worn thin, tired, and defeated with a little one on her hip. She had become a mere shadow of her once glowing self. Now it would be my turn up at-bat, and I was horrified to become that person with a kid on her hip, stained shirt and absent stare from lack of sleep. All of these thoughts reminded me of the story my mother told me. She said that, one day, she gathered up my siblings and asked if she should keep the baby, and they said yes; they were excited to have a little brother or sister. So, it was decided not to abort. Instead, my siblings were the ones who gave me the breath of life, and I am forever grateful to them. I imagine it was because my mother was getting sick and realized that it made it hard for her to carry another child ten years after her last child. Although I had grown to understand, it still cuts the flesh today. Because of that sickening remembrance of **LIVING** in the back of my mind, I did not want any children as the whole process scared me.

I often daydreamed about the opposite situation, picturing myself never being here and then thinking of now. Drearily, I thought about having a child and chatting with friends like a watchful bird dipping a spoon into pureed fruit and spooning bananas into a demanding baby bird's gaping beak. As I do this, the baby bird squawks unendingly for more banana food. It's frightening bulbous, black, swollen eyes made baby bird strain for a glimpse of me to seal me in its memory as its mother. Ugh! I would laugh at myself later for thinking this way. My imagination was always in high gear. It was my turn all right; only I was someone who could not be crossed off my own; *Dump yourself off my good buddy list*, I thought to myself. From here on out, I was stuck with myself and that someone else that had no choice but to tag along was stuck within me. I would sit and think long and hard about this new situation I found myself in which, felt more like a precarious and slippery slope of doom on an oceanic ride than a moment of happiness which, was wrong.

Comparing the beginnings of this brand new life to the one I had grown up quite accustomed to, I ignited my mind into a fevered pitch of imagining, which was where I found myself drifting into many strange and make-believe worlds on multiple occasions. Although there were many fantastical images I conjured up in my mind, I always had a colorful imagination that took real-life situations and turned them into something wild and untamed.

What was this foreign thing growing inside of me? Incubators-R-Us had come calling on my body, and as that thought was percolating, Tchaikovsky's "Dance of the Sugar Plum Fairy" would begin to play in my mind. I envisioned sugar plum termites dancing around me, the sugar plum queen termite shitting out egg after egg right in tune with the music. Clad in tutus sprinkled in fairy dust and sporting tiaras on their big heads, my termites in waiting would click their long-jointed legs together and dance macabre dances while waving their magic wands towards me. As this played out in my mind, I envisioned an undulating abdomen delivering thousands of egg babies to the termite maids in waiting. Disgusted by the mental image of myself, I sat down on the sofa to clear my thoughts. Then, oddly enough and clearly overtaking my emotions, a feeling lurked somewhere in the dim, cobwebbed recesses of my mind and rushed forward.

From this, I emerged with a faint twinge of excitement which sat me upright from my reclining position on the couch. *Could this be what my calling had been? Why would it be a child?* I didn't want it to be. I had such a terrible childhood; I would not know the first thing about giving a child a beautiful life. My life was changing in so many ways that I had not planned for me. I didn't know what to do with myself, and I was quite confused about the whole thing. I had so many questions that I could not answer, and I felt frightened and insecure yet once again in my life. With no mother to turn to and no sisters close to sit and chat with, there again arose that familiar fear of the girl who was tired of drifting on the sea of life, and who was now in the throes of life, being tumbled about in the waves of uncertainty again. I didn't like that feeling, and I definitely did not like the new turn of events that were happening to me.

Thinking back to a few months earlier of the tearful moment when I stood in the doorway of my empty condo flashed through my mind. I saw myself there on the landing, gripping the door-knob to my beloved home for the last time, and I recalled how much it hurt. But recalling the past made me start to see the beginnings of what was a bigger picture in progress. The day I closed the door to my condo was the day that I began to close the door on that singular and selfish chapter in my life. The chapter where I thought I knew everything there was to know about everything there was to know, yet I knew nothing about everything there *was* to know about everything…even love, until after the birth of my first child. My imagination completely controlled me and forever fed the fire that burned with a dark red light in my heart by bringing me a plethora of dreams. With my wild imagination, a big heart, and a tortured soul, I felt that dark fantasy, love, fear, and horror were in my blood.

That brought me back to those frightening events I endured as a young girl. Recounting it made the pain ease a bit but still made me cry. I had to get out of the slump I resided in.

I begin to love this creature and to anticipate her birth as a fresh twist to a knot which I don't wish to untie.

~Mary Wollstonecraft~

5

The T*Ruth* about Ruth

Between the 1940s and '70s, women with particular circumstances of problematic pregnancies would sometimes be prescribed a synthetic form of estrogen, known as Diethylstilbestrol, or DES, to prevent a miscarriage. Mama was one of those women who were prescribed this medication while pregnant, and I the recipient. As I grew, Mama always took care of informing me of the dangers I might potentially face as a DES daughter in basic terms as I became a young girl. However, she never made mention of (from what I can recall), any information about an incompetent cervix to me. Looking back, I realize now that I was too small to have such complicated conversations and can probably only remember the basics of what she told me, and never told me what she didn't know herself. When I started my period at age eleven, it was determined by physicians that I would undergo pap smears every six months to ensure I did not have any abnormalities of the cervix that could lead to cervical cancer.

What I know now is that women who are born to mothers who took DES are not only at risk for cervical cancer but for a whole host of other issues as well as an incompetent cervix during their own pregnancies. An incompetent cervix can dilate before the pregnancy is full-term, resulting in miscarriage or premature birth. I hadn't even given the dangers of Diethylstilbestrol any real thought during my pregnancy as issues. That was, until one morning as I laid in bed stretching and getting ready for the day to begin.

Joey had left early for work, and I woke to the warm rays of the sun streaming in the window. The sun felt wonderful, and being able to sleep in for the first time in a long time felt even better. Wanting to do my lazy cat routine and lounge for a while in the bed and stretch, I lifted my arms above my head and pointed my feet down, preparing to stretch every muscle in my body. Suddenly, there was a strange sensation, a pop somewhere deep inside me, which stunned me for a second, and then stunned me again as I felt the warmth spread between my thighs. Still stunned, I wasn't sure what was happening, and then the realization hit me that there was blood gushing and spilling out of me and onto the sheets. Fear came calling out of every pore in my body, marking its territory while roaming freely in my mind. If fear had a scent, it would be the scent of the glands of a wild beast marking its territory because it held me terrified in its grip, ready to move in for the kill after stalking its prey. Making my way carefully out of bed, all I could think of was losing the child I was carrying. I, afraid to get up, knew I must try and stem the bleeding, and so I made my way to the bathroom, concerned about how I was going to get help since I was all alone in the house. I couldn't think straight; no one was home; even most of the neighbors were away at work. Blood, more blood, the sight of blood pouring down my legs and onto the floor told me that the baby inside of me was not going to be with me for much longer. I sat down on the toilet and cried as huge clots fell into the toilet stool. Then, without any more hesitation, I threw open the bathroom window and screamed for help as I grew more frightened by the sight of my own blood. Thankfully, a neighbor who had not left for work yet heard my cries for help and came over, letting herself in with the spare key, and called both an ambulance and Joey. The ambulance arrived quickly, and right behind them was Joey, frightened and confused about what was happening. On the way to the hospital, I confided to the EMT sitting with me that I was sure I was no longer pregnant. Seeing the large clump of blood at the bottom of the stool, he told me that a miscarriage may have occurred, and the thought of what I would have to tell Joey made my heart very unhappy. However, once I was in the examining room, an ultrasound was performed. Resting quite peacefully on the lining of the uterus was my baby, safe and sound inside the womb. I smiled at what I saw on the screen, swearing to myself that I could make out hands clasped behind the head and one leg crossed over the other in true beach style, lying on a raft in the middle of my Pacific Ocean. This baby is going to be a fighter because it was wrought from the sea and placed inside me. God performs miracles on every level, far beyond anything I would ever be able to comprehend, as much as I had never wanted children because of my own childhood. The thought of losing the precious life growing inside of me was more than I could fathom. Then the question of how I was going to maintain this pregnancy to term became a very real and frightening prospect, and that scared me. My worries were not over; a week later I was still lightly bleeding, which was a source of concern for the doctors who determined it to be due to an incompetent cervix caused by my DES exposure while in utero. Of course, this was a shock to me as I had never heard of such a thing. They explained that there would be no way to maintain my pregnancy without a cerclage, a procedure that sewed the cervix closed to keep my baby inside.

The doctor informed me that a cerclage would be better because we didn't want a miscarriage to happen.

The cerclage was the straightforward part, the hard part would be the bedrest that was to stem the bleeding, and with five more months of pregnancy to go, uphill seemed much more like a mountain to climb. Now, more than ever, with the reality of what lay ahead of me to bring this pregnancy to term, I felt hemmed down by my new surroundings, and the girl I once knew and loved grew further and further away from my present self and into my remote past.

That girl had faded into a distant era with the words "fade to black" tattooed on her forehead. In my wildest imagination, I sadly watched my old self sinking to the bottom of the personal lake that resides in all of our souls, while the new me tried to rescue her. But it didn't manifest. Her chiffon nightgown twirled weightlessly about her colorless limbs, all the while she peered back at me with unseeing, unblinking eyes. How frightening it is to say goodbye to your old self. One of her arms was outstretched as if she (me) were grasping for the past as she sank, waving a cadaverous goodbye to her photo-negative twin, me. TIME separated her from me, making the process of being and becoming someone new, to be terrifying. TIME mentally and physically disjointed me from my old perception of self. The new gravity of the situation I was in with the passing of each monotonous day seemed as if it would never change. Although it was a trying task to part with my old belief system in many ways, my stubborn new self fought for a place in my life.

Joey did his best to keep me entertained, and there were some evenings where he would sit and I would recline, both with our long lists of prospective names for our new baby. So, we would compare and discuss. I would cross out some names; he would put stars next to others, and ultimately, both of us would agree to disagree. We had found out we were having a girl who left us with one million names to choose from. Joey wanted an Italian name, and I wanted an old-fashioned one, but no matter how many times we cross-referenced each other's list, we could never agree. One evening we settled on a name that Joey came up with spontaneously, and that name was Ruth. I thought it was beautiful and was the version of the biblical story of Ruth and her mother-in-law, as well as it *was* to be her name as was my mother's. Although not a daughter-in-law, I had been a dutiful daughter, and I held fast in my faith that this child would be the same.

Finally, after months of bed rest and approximately two weeks in the hospital with my bed tilted, head down, and feet in the air, to prolong the pregnancy, Ruth made her entrance into the world a month earlier than expected, but the good news was that she was healthy, and that was all that mattered to me. The perfect forming of her tiny being coupled with the randomness of nature was no accident, and I thank God for allowing me to bear witness to His miracle of life through the robust birthing process.

Her birth was a beautiful yet confounding moment in time as I was able to witness firsthand the wonder of childbirth; however, there were still mixed emotions coursing inside me that I was having great difficulty sorting through. On one hand, I was thrilled that I had a new life to care for and love, but on the other hand, I was tired, didn't want to be bothered, and just wanted to roll over and sleep undisturbed. I didn't want the nurses coming in and out; I didn't want the baby to cry; I didn't want to change her diaper; I didn't want to feed her. Yet, on the positive side, giving birth was a beautiful experience. So, I did everything that needed to be done even though I thought I didn't want to. I knew it was the right thing to do, and I knew I had to or else. But then I didn't want anyone else touching her or taking care of her, so I put her in the bed beside me the first night of her life, and there she slept, tucked away in the hollow of my arm in my hospital bed. Periodically during the night, my eyes were open to still glance at her, making sure she was okay, peacefully sleeping next to me. The lyrics to Aerosmith's "I Don't Want to Miss a Thing" were words I was saying over and over in my mind as I watched her because I simply didn't want to miss a thing about her. I couldn't wait to bring her home and begin my new life! By that point, I found feeding, changing, and crying to be something I wanted to do.

When that day arrived, and to my surprise, Joey had gone all out, having a sign delivered to our home with all her vital statistics placed on it, announcing our new blessing to the world. We were proud parents living together with our family histories into a new and exciting chapter. The first few days at home were lovely, and I didn't get much rest as the excitement of having a new addition to the family can be such a wonderful and celebratory period of time. After all the mumblings and groaning in the past about not wanting to have children, I found myself becoming mesmerized by every inch of her. Ten fingers, ten toes, fat legs, little nose. Staring into her sleeping face, I felt that this kid stuff might not be so bad, but I would have to come to grips with that if she kept crying in the middle of the night waking me up. The final determination would be how I would end up settling into motherhood. The jury was still out on it all, and I would have to wait a few more weeks until I was delirious from lack of sleep to really make my final decision about this baby stuff.

I questioned my own feelings about motherhood, wondering how I could be missing the sim card that made women want to pin funny little barretts in the baby's hair. Who was this mysterious person from above that reached down, placing a sim card in my mind to program it? I looked at Ruth's twenty pounds of hair that looked more like a bonnet of curls, her newborn skin, and eyelashes that rested upon her alabaster face. Although still reserved about my own feelings, there was one thing I knew, and that was that she was beautiful. It wasn't her; it was me that was afraid of it all.

The truth to be told was that I had always felt more like a man than a woman when it came to wanting to be a mom and care for a child, and I didn't want the "her" responsibilities placed squarely upon my shoulders. Enviously, I watched Joey come and go freely as I used to, but now I was weighed down. He slept through the night like I used to, but now I had to get up when she cried in the night. He got himself dressed as I used to; now I got two people dressed. He ate unimpeded as I used to; I now juggled eating with one hand and cooking for three people. His household chores went on as usual, and mine did, too, only now I had to cart around a sack of potatoes on my hip as I performed my duties. When we made plans to leave the house, he got himself ready as I used to; now I got the baby ready, the bottle ready, the diaper bag ready, then myself ready all the while being rushed because I inevitably ran late. It was a new life, one I wasn't so sure of, and I wondered if that was what the dream was all about. If it was, I was ungrateful for the life sentence. However, I hoped the baby was dreaming little dreams of me. This chain-gang shit was for the birds. I didn't like breaking big rocks (pregnancy), into little rocks (babies), but the reality of it all was that I was in my own creative presence, wearing prison stripes. I did not have the grit nor the strength nor the get up and go to pull myself out of my funk and see how wonderful and beautiful all of this was. With all that said, make no mistake, I loved this baby girl, and the love I held for her, tied in a knot I would never untie.

Giving birth to your first child is the closest you can ever come to magic.

~Unkown~

You can't put your feet on the ground until you've touched the sky.

~**Paul Auster**~

ODE TO A WINTER PRINCESS
(Ruth)

Sweetest little angel of mine
Fragile in every way,
You quietly stole into my life
One cold, grey winter's day

Your skin as fair as alabaster
Hair as black as night
The winter queen she kissed your cheeks
Then blessed me with your sight.

You are her child, this much is true
With demeanor cool in measure
An icy appearance can be deceiving
And masks a hidden treasure

The queen she buried her treasure chest
Inside your beating heart
Then tossed away the snowflake key
So her gift would never depart

Within your soul lies warmth and love
And caring beyond the north,
For you possess the winter's promise
The new sun to be born

Your heart beats true and deep within
You guard her magic poultice deep
It is beyond my wildest dream
But secures her while she sleeps

I know now that the gift of you
Is beyond my wildest notion
You are my sun, and I your planet
B'yond forever you have my devotion

KC

6

Soles

As previously stated, sleep and dreams have never been a part of my nightly repertoire, although experts say we all dream quite often. I rarely, if ever, have been able to say, "I had a crazy dream last night." The lunar landscape of the little sleep I got kept me from remembering anything at all unless it was vivid. Instead, there was a burning dryness in my mind that gave me nothing to report back to earth about the following morning, except static snow on a screen from the night before. If in fact I do dream, I simply cannot recall things most do. As well, sleeping has always been a hard-won nightly battle my entire life, as a thousand and one nights have been spent sharing the company of hours on the clock face as the hands moved "round" and "round," waving at me in their prison. The second hand ticked by as my anxiety grew, and I counted the last hours of sleep of what I had left until the alarm clock would blare in the morning. The scarlet second hand reminded me of the danger of little sleep.

Whenever these nights would haunt me, and they were more often than not, I think back to my favorite set of sheets as a child. They were sheets covered with Snoopy, Charlie Brown, and Lucy, all with the speech bubbles coming from their mouths with words of wisdom for the young mattress dweller. I cherished every saying on the speech bubble sheets from the Peanuts gang because they, as children, had such an ideal life with lots of friends that I would have liked. They lived in a great neighborhood and shared what seemed like wonderful holidays together, complete with the best part that I could ever wish for, friends, lots of them. My special sheets had one saying in particular from Charlie Brown that made me long for a great night's sleep as a little girl. His words of wisdom were, "Happiness is waking up and discovering you still have two hours of sleep left." How I would wish I could go back to sleep should I wake up in the middle of the night. I would stare at that image on the sheets and hope for drowsiness. However, if I had gotten up to use the bathroom or just been jarred out of sleep for no reason at all, sleep had left my soul. Falling back to sleep rarely happened gracefully, no matter how hard I besieged God for help in sleeping. Instead, I would just lay there and toss and turn for hours staring back-and-forth between the "o'clock's" and the sheets in the dark. My mother always said I was a night owl, and now in my older years, I proudly declare that I *am* a self-proclaimed hoot owl that has come to accept my inability to sleep soundly like the rest of the world. Joey, on the other hand, has the uncanny ability to sleep anywhere, anytime, anyplace, and this will be the only time I admit ever that I am fiercely jealous of his sleeping capabilities. He and I could be in the middle of a conversation after a long day of work, and before you know it, poof! His eyes drooped, his neck rocked to and fro, and he had set sail on a journey into La La Land as I jabbered on, unaware he was sitting, rocking his sleep in tunes of saws and rasps. Once I realized he was no longer paying attention to me and sleeping instead, it drove me to the brink of madness because of his ability to drift off so easily into the land of nod, transitioning from the world of awareness to being out like a light instantaneously.

On one particular evening after another futile conversation in bed, I did my usual tossing and turning for an hour or so and then finally drifted off to sleep and found myself in a predicament that I knew required me to hide. If not, it would be a matter of life or death and all I could feel from the situation I found myself in was that I was frightened, I needed to take my little magical sprite Ruth with me and run.

Oh gosh, I'm scared, and I've got to run! I heard myself think. "Come, Ruth, let Mommy pick you up because we have to hide! Hang on to Mama, and I won't let anything hurt you." I had oozing sweat and oil from every pore in my body, and the oil and water mix dripped from my face as I frantically searched for somewhere to hide. However, it suddenly became clear that I was watching myself in a movie because everything in the picture was black and white just like the old picture shows. Oddly, I could feel every emotion going on inside the movie and could read every thought firing through my mind. It was as if I were in two places at once because I was. Was I dreaming? I must be, but I missed the part of how I got to this destination.

Outside of the movie screen, I noted I was standing in the pitch black as my eyes began to adjust to the darkness enveloping me. My surroundings became clearer to see. I was hanging on to my magic bundled toddler because I could see that I was in a cavernous room encapsulated in a black stone that seemed to go on forever. I got the feeling that I was in space, outer space, maybe floating and maybe not, but this room was neither near Earth nor on solid ground. I was too afraid to look down, not knowing if there was a floor; the feeling I was getting was that there was nothing below me but sheer black depths of stars and nothingness that were real. This room I was in was entirely empty save for the viewing window where I stood and watched the picture show…starring me. The viewing window itself was surrounded by cool, black stone and a counter that surrounded the room with this material as well. Below the screen was a shelf on which I could rest my elbows. I was alone in the dark room but didn't feel threatened or afraid to be in my surroundings. The only fear I felt was at what I was witnessing on the screen and seeing my daughter and me inside that viewing window. What I saw playing before me was a film, complete with the black bands at the top and bottom of the screen and the sound old films made when they slipped in their frames and flapped about until someone fixed it.

The only two people recognizable so far in the film were Ruth and I, and I could see that we were alone in a large and deserted city. I stared wide-eyed at the scene before me and became a frightened, gladiatorial spectator, sensing real danger as I cheered myself on. Adrenaline pumping, I wanted to know what my own outcome would be. Anticipation whipped my eyes that were transfixed on the window because fear was coursing through my veins while wondering what I might see. The intense fear I was experiencing in the film translated from one dimension into another as it tore into my own psyche and nerve receptors like an explosion of an adrenaline rush. Grasping Ruth to my chest, I could actually feel the reason everything was black and white in the world because the information radiated through my body, neurons provided me with communication information that I needed to know about because of what I was seeing. The color of life has been drained from the world, leaving all the shades of black and white to filter their way through everything that was left on earth. Just as it electronically filtered information through my brain via the electric highway, with every heartbeat, it crept into the calcified crevices of mortar, bricks, mood, and mind.

It lingered in the nightmarish lunar landscapes of all of our worst imaginings. How fitting this was as black-and-white or clear-cut colors that defined or mirrored so many aspects of our lives seemed to change fluidly. Just like yin and yang, day and night, good and evil. The days had indeed become evil, and the end of time was upon us within the setting I was looking at. It was frightening to be in the viewing area of a theater while floating through the universe. How can one be in two places at the same time?! My feet sturdily in the stars, my eyes staring at the picture screen where I could feel the emotions of my being. This was because I existed at the same time inside a room and inside of the screen. Both screen and I stood face to face in the mystery of *time* and space.

Being back inside of the picture show again and guided by some mysterious force, I ran as fast as I could with Ruth. I knew instinctively not to stop, or we would not survive whatever it was that was creeping in behind us. There wasn't anything physical about this creeping threat, whether it was something of evil nature or spiritual force. A battle between good and evil encroach in on the living space of the earth. It was something that could not be contained, which was a frightening perspective on how civilization was and what it had grown to be. I was led, by what, I didn't know, to the doors of a large building and, at that point, instinctively knew that I needed to go to the **third** floor. Why the third floor and not the first? I found the **NEED** to get to the third floor, for which I took as a sign from above, and so, I followed my instincts. The Holy Trinity? A trilogy? A haiku? The sun, stars, and moon? Or was it Vini Vidi Vici? To me, all five represented the cycle of life to death. The Father was the birth of life from our creator, and the sun (son) was living your best life, and then the spirit, death of one's life where you move to a different realm. The sun and stars and moon, where the sun births life from the ground every year in this cycle, the stars represented all the wishes and dreams we pin our success to, and the moon was enlightenment and darkness when we closed our eyes for the last time. The Haiku? A pattern of three, birth and growth, first line, the second, long life, and the last line of life coming to an end so quickly, just as quickly the haiku lasts. Vini Vidi Vici? I came (arrived here on earth). I saw (the path I needed to take); I conquered (lived a strong and fruitful life that I could reflect on before death). Dripping sweat as it was hot; the air was shocked by things that could not be seen. The sun was hanging in the air like an overripe melon ready to burst and spill its seeds upon the earth. Only those seeds were not for renewal, but for sowing and then wreaking havoc. Those seeds would eventually spread roots and wreak distruction upon the land. They would not produce fruit but rather destroy it by giving birth to man's transgressions, sinfulness, and destructive ways that hurt our precious Mother Earth. The sun, usually filled with color, looked and smelled rotten despite everything else that had been written in black-and-white. I saw it as a putrid orange color as it hung there in the sky, boring holes into everything. Its damaging rays sought out for anything it could find to harm. I climbed each stair, stretching my legs to their full capacity, gasping for each breath, clogged by the vile fog and sun that had ravaged the earth of its most darling prize, oxygen. Already tapped from running and climbing stairs, I didn't have much left to give and the added weight of Ruth on my hip had tested every ounce of stamina I had.

Standing in the viewing area of the theater, it dawned on me that I was the only guest invited to this premier. Watching intently and deeply engrossed in what would happen next, my anxiety level increased while experiencing two sets of emotions into separate frames of time, my perception of real-time and the manufactured time on the screen. Sweat was already dripping from my face out of fear.

Inside the picture show, my eyes adjusted to the light in the barren room, and I saw that the floor of the building I had been used as a classroom in the past. The old-fashioned desks were askew in the room, making it seem as though the occupants of those seats had left in a hurry. As quiet as I possibly could, I moved a desk in between two windows so that Ruth and I could not be seen from the street below. I gently clasped my hand around her mouth and motioned with one finger to my lips to keep silent. My lungs screamed for oxygen as I struggled to breathe yet I could not make any noise for fear of being heard.

Inside the viewing arena, I was also covered with sweat by the fear I was feeling inside the picture show. It isn't every day you watch yourself waiting for the Lord himself to return and call his faithful home. I had time to reflect on the picture show and came to the conclusion that this was a metaphor of sorts for the evil that is abundant in the world, and the difficulty believers have in attempting to avoid the pitfalls of those temptations. I, too, included.

"Ruth," I whispered, "please don't make any noise; you must sit as still as a *winter's* day," I peek, peek, peeked cautiously out of the window, barely able to contain my fear. Nothing, nothing, nothing, not a breeze, breeze, nor a shimmer off the pavement below. Not a movement to be seen, and then I heard it, a trumpet or horn of some unearthly tone, sounded from above. It then changed into an earthly sound so beautiful that its tone resonated through everything left in the world. "Ruth," I whispered, "please don't make any noise. You must sit as still as a *summer's* day." I peeked, peeked, peeked, cautiously out of the window, barely able to contain my fear. Again, nothing, nothing, nothing, not even a movement, movement, nor a human sound, with nothing to be seen and then I heard it again. The trumpet or horn of some sort sounded from above and operated on an unearthly wave through my body. The horn sounded once again yet sent out a beautiful song by its tone and resonance. It was announcing the return of the great creator himself. I stood at my post in the darkness, watching from the viewing window all the while, my heart pounding and face sweating while gripping the edge of the marble in heightened anticipation of what was going to happen. Would I make it down in time with Ruth? I became afraid of what I might see next.

"Let's go, Ruth!" I shouted. "Hang on tight; Mama's got to run!" I navigated the stairwell with Ruth on my hip and then jumped, taking two stairs at a time and then the last three all at once to make it down to the street, and then sprinted out of the front door and onto the open road. *Where did all these people come from? They must have been hiding like me. I've got to run if I'm going to catch up with everyone,"* I thought to myself. I started running with the crowd, running, running, running, panting, panting for air. I see people being lifted; they were flying, floating…being taken home. Up, up, and away…I count the number of the soles of shoes rising above my head. Two, four, six…And I note that there aren't many people being caught up. *Am I going?* I wondered nervously from the viewing area and began to root myself on with the anticipation that squeezed my insides tight like an octopus grasping at me. Tears began streaming down my face as prayers flowed freely asking to see what it was that I wanted to see.

"We are almost there!" I said to Ruth as I ran along with the crowd. I knew it would only be a second until we both got caught. In the movie, my face was pointed towards the sky. Only standing in the viewing area, I could not see beyond that aggravating black band above the screen that blocked my view. I watched as the soles of shoes drifted into the blackness of the screen; people's hands were outstretched, waiting for their turn to go home to heaven. I stared intently into my own face as I watched and felt the excitement and worry that was plaguing me inside the screen. There were no longer soles or souls to be seen. What about me? The picture showed the viewing screen had FADED TO BLACK...and the rest of the night I slept quite restlessly.

The next morning, the first emotion I experienced was fear, and then determination set in. The determination was to fix what was wrong in my own life and to learn more about having faith no matter what that faith might look like. Faith can come in many different forms, and it is the believer's unwavering devotion to believing without seeing that we still have good will to others. Serving mankind with love is truly the secret to great wealth in life. Ultimately, it is the richness of spirit that brings a soul to peace, and I wanted a slice for myself, as well as some magic. I needed fixing of myself, but I didn't realize it. Giving birth to my first child was her way of not only saving me but realizing the gift of magic. For her, every day was like magic to me. That made me fully aware of the dream.

The message I received from this dream was to get myself right in this life of mine. I never found out how the dream ended, if I went up, or if I were on the first bus or not. Or if I had to wait for the late bus to come and get me later due to after-school detention. Or maybe there were no more buses destined for heaven. There was one thing I didn't know, and that was that I did not want to find out firsthand. I wanted to catch the first bus home, and so I whispered a little prayer. "Lord, I do not want to be left behind, so would you please help me to open my eyes and heart to you, as you have revealed yourself to me. I want to be on the first bus, Father, and I want to sit right behind the driver so that I don't miss my stop." I guess walking towards that bus would be of great honor in order to get my feet up into the sky.

I'm a strong believer in everything is meant to be for a reason.

~Nicole Scherzinger~

7

S.S. FAITH SETS SAIL

When I was a little girl, there was never a defining moment when the realization dawned on me that we were an extremely poor family. Being poor seemed to be an unspoken rule of thumb that was just the status quo in the family. Nor did it ever dawn on me that we were poorer than the average person. And it never needed to be said; it was an unspoken truth. Us kids never asked for anything out of the ordinary because it was never going to materialize. We struggled with the day-to-day things that any family will struggle with when there is no father around with a mother who is recovering from open heart surgery. Struggles like no food, no electricity, no clothing, no money. Every ride was a bumpy one, and every corner a sharp curve. I never knew what led to the next step. As I grew older, I suppose it was those moments that solidified in my young adult mind that being a child was not cool, nor fine, instead, for me, the message was that being a child was frightening and spooky.

Childhood was not ideal, to look like those Norman Rockwell pictures I saw hanging in the welfare doctor's offices. Those kinds of lives were make-believe to me, but if they were real, they were reserved for kids with cowlicks and freckles. Just like Dick and Jane who had everything that I did not. Dick wore jeans in his world and lived on a street where there were dads who wore brimmed hats and suits to work every day. They lived on the street where there were kids who owned dogs named Spot; they flew kites and had a shiny red wagon with the words Radio Flyer emblazoned on the sides. They lived on the street where even little girls, unlike me, had things I could only dream of. Dollies had bows and pretty dresses and little girls' mommies wore high-heeled shoes, never looked frazzled, and never ever had to have heart surgery. That was a place for names like Sally and Mary, Papa, and cats that were named Bubblegum.

Nope, not in our little pink house at 1010 West 10th Street on our side of the tracks in Merced in the 1960s before our move to San Diego. There were no Dick and Janes. There were only Tyrones, Ophelias, Billys, Randalls, and Keishas. Instead, within the realms of my universe, we were *those kinds* of people who lived on the wrong side of the tracks where migrant workers, drunks, and those who didn't have a pot to piss in or a window to throw it out of. There were no wagons at all, and dogs were not pedigrees named Spot but, instead, mutts who had names like Spook with only three legs and chained up in backyards to be fed chicken bones. When the mutts weren't chained, they hobbled down the street foraging for leftovers in the alleyways and baring their teeth at strangers who happened by. We lived on the street where there *might* be a man, but not many dads. Some jobs but not much money, and plenty of moms in shifts and housecoats. They wore fuzzy slippers and pink sponge rollers in their hair that was eternally tied up with a hair rag. These were moms who were frazzled at trying to keep up a household and running on welfare checks for commodities they received once a month. Yes, we were *those* people who were like the powdered milk-drinking butts of jokes. Because of those living conditions, I wished I could be a well-smoked cigarette cast away into the gutters of busy streets only to bear witness to the comings and goings of bustling people. I wanted to be the cigarette itself: number one, everyone desired it; and number two, it was so long and beautiful with the fire of life burning through its journey on Earth. I wanted to be desired and yearned for like those magical streets I saw every time my mother drove me through them to visit the doctor. If lucky enough, when I was pulled out from the pack of cigarettes, my essence would curl around the heads of smokers as they got their fix from my addictive nature. All I wanted was to be like the others I saw and read about and could only dream of what life would be like as it was a volatile time in life to be a bi-racial child.

When she was alive, I would ask Mom questions about the future and attempt to figure out how to escape our poverty and become something as fancy as a smoker living on the other side of the tracks. I would not only be able to save myself but her as well when I grew up. My questions were those usual questions a little kid would ask their parents, and I would ask her what she thought I should be when I grew up. I knew what she wanted to be, but hearing her dreams for me always made for a pleasant conversation. Mama would often tell me that the future was something that one could not predict no matter how hard it was planned for because life already had plans for us. She always wanted to be a pilot, but in her time, women were not doing things like that. So I suppose her advice was coming from her heart because of her own yearnings that fell through the cracks. I supposed she was enamored with Amelia Earhart and wanted to do that as well, be a pilot. The best thing to do, she would say, is to always be prepared in life spiritually. Mama was a devout Catholic and believed that faith should be the framework of life and the hallmark of an individual. Although we did not have the perfect image of a family that the church believed in, she made sure we were immersed in its religious teachings. However, over the span of many years of defeats and disappointments, the winds of time loosened my moorings and set me adrift from the shoreline of faith I had been raised in.

After having that particular dream I had, it was clear that mama's past advice was needed once again to be central in my life. The message revealed would need to become a focal point that I could use to strengthen my belief system in order to cultivate and harvest the life I wanted. Faith needed to be the platform I could stand on, like an island in an endless sea. I had been drifting aimlessly in this life for too long, bottom-feeding off of my own fears and insecurities and drawing negative power from my own shortcomings. Those shortcomings would then manifest into lesions and boils from which would spur on the fears even more. Now, there was a little one whom I loved more than life itself, and she had become the keel on what was fast developing into a sleek and better-designed sailing craft named Faith. Gone was the rickety dinghy that continually took on water; now in its place was a vessel complete with rigging and lifeboats and one gal, semi-experienced to be the whole crew.

Hello? I'm working on being the best that I can be. I hope you are proud of me; I guess life leads you to its plans, and everything that happens must be meant to be.

If the sight of the blue skies fills you with joy,
If a blade of grass springing up in the fields has power to move you,
if the simple things of nature have a message that you understand,
Rejoice, for your soul is alive.

~ Eleonora Duse ~

8

A Tree for Prayers, Boo-Boos, and Cake

A few weeks after having another dream, pregnancy came my way once again. This time, it was an exciting punctuation mark that meant so much to me. Now that there was another child on the way, it was high time to move from the age of the three-family home and into new digs around the corner and down the road to a lovely street named Grandview Avenue. I marveled at how life had a way of bringing things full circle and will or will not break the connection. Several years back when I was single, I had looked to purchase a house on the very same street we were now moving to.

That house was about six houses away from the home we were going to live in. In the new house's backyard, there was a beautiful tree. There were limbs that stretched out like an umbrella. It appeared as if the previous owner had maintained and cared for it well because it was a gracious and magnificent tree. I'm not sure what it is about trees for me, but they have a magic spell about them. Their big and gracious boughs blowing gently in the wind made me marvel at their beauty. I really admired the house I looked at while single, but knowing it was too much house for a single girl, I passed it by. Instead, I settled on my beautiful condo in New Haven, which turned out to be much more manageable for me. Now here I was, several years later, back on Grandview Avenue. Only this time toting a family. This time around, I was getting an even better house than before.

God works in mysterious ways, I thought to myself pulling into the driveway and smiling at this really cool coincidence. This particular house had stayed empty for twelve years and was in need of some repair, but the house had tremendous bones, making it a wonderful place to raise our children. It was at the top of a hill, and I could see for miles from this perch. The house overlooked a lovely little park for kids to come and play basketball, and nearby was an elementary school where I could hear children playing at recess time. The grounds around the house were beautiful, with flowering dogwood trees and bushes scattered about in the new yard. Although the grounds had been neglected, once spruced up they would provide hours of respite in the cool evenings.

Behind the house and next to the driveway grew that large, beautiful tree moving gently in the wind. Admiring it for its beauty, one could understand nature's message and gift while staring at it. I could almost imagine each individual leaf as a tiny and very grateful hand applauding through its branches making me realize it was much more important than myself in this world of ours. Each graceful motion of the leaves was like the tree itself giving thanks for our lives and praising the unseen force for creating them. This particular tree gave me automatic solace when I looked at it, and as I stood underneath it and placed my hands upon its bark, it made me rejoice in being in touch with nature. With that, it was decided that this tree would be my prayer tree at this new home, a place where I could go to seek comfort, pray, and talk to God. Whereas the outside of the house was a delight and brought such peace to me, the inside was a completely different story. The house needed work, work, and more work.

Although there wasn't major work to be done, a home always represented something sacred and beautiful. In my adult life, every place I have ever lived has had to have a special place to use for my retreat, a place where I could go to find quiet, meditate, and or have respite from the daily grand mysteries that have a way of giving so much to me without taking anything in return. For instance, the sound the wind makes when it blows through a tree is like the rhythmic sound of the ocean beating back and forth from the shore on a calm day. When leaves moved after twelve years of neglect, they did their best to attract attention. There was also updating that needed to be accomplished before the house could be lived in once again. One of the tasks at hand was rehabbing the kitchen before the birth of our second child, and as a result of that, the bed, dining room table, refrigerator, and trash container ended up in the living room alongside Ruth and I who couldn't do much more than sit in a chair and watch everything take place. Every ounce of household chores that needed to happen during that particular time became a time within the confines of the living room. Not only did I have to attempt to put together meals in the living room, but I also had to wash dishes in the bathtub we didn't use. That particular bathroom was on the other side of the house, and I had to bring them back to the living room to put them away. I was thoroughly disgusted. As construction continued, tension grew, and I felt pinned into one room with a chair in a very large house where I would nap made me love this old chair. This chair was old and low to the ground, and it was a chair with much-needed work to be done when the house was finished; the wallpaper still needed to be hung, and decorations needed to happen before the birth of this baby. The chair in the living room that had been left behind by the previous owners that had moved out so long ago. I wondered why they would leave with twelve years' worth of dust on it looking lonely and abandoned with no one to love it. It was a pathetic chair, so I decided that I would love it and would use it to sit in during the day when I grew tired. The fabric had to have been a throwback from the thirties. It was blue and white and green, a sickening green, like the color of moss growing on the back of a sloth in the depths of a jungle. The floral design on it was reminiscent of some designer's attempts at a contemporary design that failed miserably, and yet I still loved this little chair. The side of the chair had been shredded by an unknown cat that would sharpen his claws to a dangerous point. Probably in contempt of the awful fabric, but the cat was no longer here, most likely long dead. Maybe that cat's name was Bubblegum. And that is how the awful chair got its official name, the Cat Chair. I would tell Ruth that I was going to take a nap in the Cat Chair and that she should not go anywhere while I did. I would explain to her that Mama was tired because her big belly made her sleepy, and she would shake her head as if she understood, go get her toys, and plop down beside me. The Cat Chair was comfortably oversized and fit me just right as I sat there sleeping, big belly protruding out in front of me, and my head rolled back. That scene looking like an oversized Goldilocks trying to find the chair that fits just right. Maybe there's a chair that would have never held up under the weight of me; Mama Bear's chair would've been too tight, but would Papa Bear's chair hold me just fine at this late stage in my pregnancy? As I dozed in the comfortable midday sun, Ruth would play at my feet, but I was only half asleep, and I would periodically gaze at her with one bleary eye to make sure she was still there.

She was always good like that, never straying away from me no matter where I was or what I was doing. If she wasn't by my side, she spent time at a neighborhood daycare, where she could play with other kids her age, and I could go to school. This gave me some free time to run errands and attend doctors' appointments that I needed to keep. One appointment I particularly looked forward to was going to have an ultrasound done which would determine the sex of the baby. My ultrasound appointment had been something I looked forward to in both pregnancies as I wanted to know the sex of the baby so that I could plan accordingly.

I was never good at surprises, and I did not want to wait to find out the sex of the baby I was carrying. However, these ultrasound technicians seemed as if they weren't quite sure about the sex of the baby. During the procedure, I heard one technician second-guessing herself, and she said to the other technician, "A shy XY?" She was questioning if she was seeing a boy or not, and what did that mean? A shy XY? Why were they not sure of the sex, or they just couldn't get a good enough peek? I didn't question her about her hesitant re-action; instead, I waited for her to determine what it was that she was seeing, and soon she confirmed that I would be having a son. With that wonderful news, I went on my way excited to deliver the good news to my family. Ruth was as happy as a toddler could be about the arrival of a sibling, sometimes understanding and some-times clinging to me like I was going to leave her. So, to help her along she and I spent a lot of time together planning ways to prepare for the upcoming arrival of her little brother. She and I would talk about his arrival as we shopped for his bedding and clothing that I would need, and I would take the time to tell her how special she was to me. She and I enjoyed spending that time together and de-cided that we would pick a beautiful blue blanket for her little brother that was coming. It was nice to get away from the house with each other because the house left us with little to no privacy during the daytime hours, so just to get away as mother and daugh-ter was more than I could've asked for. Joey was thrilled about the son he was going to have, and once again, we set about picking names, this time settling on Biagio Giuseppe for another solid Italian name to add to our family, and for my love of Shakespeare.

We talked to Ruth about her becoming a big sister to her little brother. He would be coming soon. As the arrival time came closer, we took her shopping so she could pick out a gift for him. She would ask what he was doing in my stomach, and I would have to explain to her that he was sleeping in there, but when I would say that to her, she would shake her head no, like I didn't understand what she was asking me. Those little moments that had been spent together talking about the baby were precious ones because it would be the last time that she and I would be just a twosome, just mother and daughter. Once Biagio arrived, we would grow into a "family of four," and my little girl and I would have another little person in our exclusive little club. There would be no more girls' club, as we called it, because brother was coming into the family dynamic that would change upon his arrival in the world. There are those who swear that children are directly wired to, or still have connections to heaven. I am one of those people, and Ruth is one of those kids. As a toddler, she would never stop her talking to Jesus or see her balls of light that she said she could see and even be named. Then, as the pregnancy progressed, came the time when she would lay on my stomach, one little ear straining to listen to her sibling. She would lay on my stomach for half-hour stretches listening, listening, listening, to hear; and I was never quite sure she was old enough to really express herself. I would ask Ruth, "What are you doing?" During this time; she would sometimes tell me she wanted to know what the baby was doing in there. But most of the time she would tell me she was listening to the baby sing to her. After she was done listening, she would get up and say, "Mama, baby not a boy, baby a girl. She has a boo-boo, and she smells like cake." Then she would walk off and begin to play with her toys. It wasn't just one time she told me that, it was many times, over and over and over. She was insistent, insistent, insistent, that the baby was a girl and that the baby had a boo-boo. The boo-boos part of what she said gave me shivers up and down my spine because her little face was so matter-of-fact. However, I would laugh it off in my adult ways just like any big person would laugh at a little kid when they say something so far out. Her words would scare me the most. I would tell Joey what she said, and he would tell me not to worry. Then we would make light of the cake part, wondering what it was that she thought she smelled that was so sweet. Joey would jokingly say he was sure it wasn't me that she smelled because I had not cleaned out my belly button since the invention of hand soap, and we would laugh our asses off.

But then, Cake. The baby smells like a cake would always creep slowly back into my mind. It was creepy and curious but cute. Curious but more likely a creepy kind of cute. I could picture in the *Twilight Zone* sort of way. Ruth never stopped insisting that the baby was a girl who had a boo-boo. It seemed to possess her as an obsession to take over an entire portion of someone's life. She would tell me every day the baby was sick, that the baby had a boo-boo, and that the baby smelled like cake. She even wanted to name the baby "Cake." Those declarations scared me, and I would tell her the baby was fine. Her brother would be just fine, but when I spoke those words, she would just blankly stare back at me with her large, knowing eyes. When I tucked to her in bed at night, the last thing she would say before she dropped off in slumber was that she couldn't wait to see her baby Cake, and I would smile at her, thinking to myself of that date in May would be the one where she would see her baby Cake. And I would worry, thinking to myself that Cake was never going to come because, at this point, she told me every day the baby was sick, that the baby had a boo-boo, and that the baby smelled like cake. I was two weeks late, two weeks overdue, couldn't breathe, and just plain anxious for his arrival. I was happy with this child, yet physically miserable, and more than ready than ever to have this cake. I couldn't wait to be able to enjoy this new addition to the family and get the frightening predictions of my silly but also sweet two-year-old reigned in.

Ode to a Celestial Child

I'm sure the sun did pierce my womb
And kiss your tiny face
She wrapped you in her warmest rays
And gave you love's embrace.

When you began your journey here
To walk the many roads
I knew you'd face life's many trials
And carry many loads

How can you know this? If you dare to ask
And *how* is what I'll tell
Because the sun protected you
By bathing you in her spell

One glance upon those sun-kissed cheeks
and bronze bedazzled skin,
It's true, you're part celestial being
The sun made you her kin

A fiery disposition flows
Quite fiercely through your veins
Profusion of shimm'ry, golden locks
Crown you with a mane

Despite your burden, precious child
Despite what you must face
Despite what life has planned for you
Of fear? I see no trace

I know now that the gift of you
Is beyond my wildest notion
You are my sun and I your planet
B'yond forever you have my devotion

KC

"Birth is not only about making babies. Birth is about making mothers—strong, competent, capable mothers who trust themselves and know their inner strength."

~ **Barbara Katz Rothman** ~

9

Biagio the Beautiful?

B iagio made his entrance into the world two weeks later, and he didn't come quietly. Instead, he made a grand entrance so that the world knew he was here. Having been scheduled for a cesarean section, I couldn't be happier as Ruth was a vaginal birth that I was not yearning to repeat. But this little guy, he was big, too big for me to deliver as my hips were too small. Because of that, I wasn't complaining.

In this day and age, I couldn't figure out why a woman needed to be in pain during childbirth. Now I completely understood the health issues associated with the birthing process. The medications and delicate procedures that interfere with the natural process of birth may help, and maybe not as well. But, with that said, I could still not understand nor wrap my mind around the fact that women wanted to remain wracked in pain for hours delivering a baby. The night before the scheduled procedure, I went to bed almost giddy over the fact that this child who was two weeks late would be in the world first thing in the morning, and it would happen for me with-out pain or much distress. But, as my luck always seemed to go, it was not to be that way, as he decided to come into the world three hours before the scheduled procedure. Hard labor ensued almost immediately after the first labor pains began. My incompetent cervix was rapidly opening after being scarred shut from the previous pregnancy, and by the time I reached the hospital twenty minutes later and was examined by my doctor, my cervix had opened to six centimeters. I was now in the throes of hard labor, but it felt more like doing hard time in prison. My old buddies from the chain gang were back again insisting, this *time*, I deliver a watermelon through a hole the size of a drinking straw in record time. While this drama was playing out for me, Joey, the overseer, stood to watch over his charge, sweat dripping off his brow while attempting to give me orders on how to breathe. I wanted to slap the shit out of him or maybe bite his stomach that was pressed against my cheek at the side of the bed because I was in so much pain. After all, it was his fault I was in this mess and wanted to do something to him to inflict as much pain on him as I could so he could feel pain as well as it wasn't my fault, I was always the "innocent" one. Even though I knew better, I was making things up in my mind to make me feel better. In my mind, I laughed at myself for all those crazy thoughts coursing through my brain. I figured my wild imagination was still churning, perhaps as a deflection to what was happening at that moment. Don't get me wrong, the excitement of the new baby was overwhelming, and I couldn't wait to meet him.

Oddly enough, I had had a dream about a month earlier. It dawned on me that I had already met him. The dream carried me to the porch of our house where I was sitting, relaxing with my baby in a rocking chair, holding a child that I did not recognize. The baby, wearing soft lavender overalls and a white onesie, lifted its head and said to me with a smile, "I can't wait to meet you." The dream was so surreal that I did my best to remember what that beautiful baby looked like and could summon up in my mind a smile on its round face. So taken aback by this dream, I couldn't wait to meet Biagio either.

Back in my reality and not wanting to cause any more of a scene that was already formulated in my mind to carry out, I decided medication was the better bet. I begged for drugs and mercy, which ultimately spared Joey from his own personal hospital gurney. He kept instructing me to breathe which was annoying me, but I was trying. All I could think about was the person who came up with the notion of breathing when you are already breathing, panting, and writhing in pain. Breathing? What's the point of doing it any different than one does on a normal day? Does it automatically re-move the pain like magic? NO. And because of this, I was seriously considering all of the above, but there were many things at stake. How could I hurt the man who was the father of my child, and would I come up with more things to do to him while in labor? And so, I controlled my out of control thought process. Fear had gripped me again and whispered in my ear; reminding me of the words Ruth had said. My anticipation for this child made me a nervous mother; I hollered loudly and groveled about on the bed, calling out for an anesthesiologist or whomever would listen. There was no shame in my game at that point because pain like that is something I didn't do well with. I briefly thought about my Native Indian princess her-itage. My mom used to say that some Indian women silently gave birth and that it was a shameful thing to do to make noise while ex-periencing it. *Well,* I thought to myself, *let me scream even louder for pain medication because I am not a brave native Indian princess but a cow-ardly commoner who does not like pain and has nothing to prove to others that I could give birth like some superhero.*

And so, at the top of my lungs, I screamed in pain for drugs. Any kind, of any sort. Prescription, street, homemade, or IV. You name it, I wanted it, even if stolen. Right there, to put me out of my misery. I was like an old horse ready for the glue factory as I waited for the anesthesia. Strap me up and set me free and prepare me for the drug FAC-TO-REEEE. I was so excited I suppose the doctor must've gotten tired of my crybaby antics because I was on my way to the operating room, and an anesthesiologist appeared at the door. But truth be told, my OB/GYN had decided I could not vaginally deliver this baby even though he was well on his way, and the doctor had called an anesthesiologist herself. Upon the doctor's arrival, I promptly told him that I loved him as he approached me with his tools of the trade. He was like Felix the Cat standing there in the doorway and jilted a little jig with a big wide grin on his face that stretched from ear to ear. I was rolling around as his big silver-dollar eyes and his bag of magic tricks weaved enticingly into my view and then disappeared again. Calling and beckoning to him was that bag in the cerebral world of the psychedelic, telling me I would be riding the railway of the central nervous system. That was the transportation mode I wanted to take. I wanted to ride in the car of no pain or take a cab, a bus, or an Uber, whose price was the steepest and reserved for those who paid enough for first-class highs. Shortly after the anesthesiologist's arrival, the familiar twinge of a needle entered my back, and then there was nothing but peace. "Hallelujah!" I shouted and then laid down on the operating room table professing my undying love for Dr. Felix the Cat. I was in love with the kahuna who had taken my pain away with his western shamanism, numbing me to the realities of what it means to be on the bumpy plane of human pain. He stepped aside as Joey came into the operating room all swelled up like the Michelin Man, stuffed and trussed in his hospital garb. He sat by my side, held my hand, and then said, "Ready, set, go!" We were off to the races as the procedure got underway within minutes or so. It seemed to me painful that Biagio made his entrance into the world with the most soulful cry one could ever hear, but later, for a few brief moments, the doctor began lightly talking to those around her about what she was observing. "His penis looks a bit bent," I heard her say, and he just peed on me!" Biagio had been taken and laid down for examination. For a brief moment, I hung on the first comment she announced, but even though those tiny darts spilling forth from her mouth indelibly stuck, searing them into my brain. Recalling the words that had hit their mark in my mind, I tried to wish them to dissipate into the sterile environment around me by attempting to meditate on goodness and to push fear out of my life. All I wanted at that point was to lay eyes on my new baby boy and ignore what I had just heard. I couldn't wait to see what he looked like, and with anticipation building inside me, making me want to leave off from where I was and get a good peek at him only, I couldn't move my legs. From my vantage point, I couldn't see a thing with the hospital blue tarp draped between me and the procedure; I could only hear and attempt to unpack their commentary. Then hearing "He looks as if he's been partially circumcised" set off a cacophony of alarms in my mind. Those words spoken within earshot were like water balloons being tossed about at a party. They hit their mark with accuracy and burst, leaving the contents of those words to douse my happy moment in fear. However, the excitement of this moment in time took the gravity and weight of those words spoken and burned them inside me like a smoldering piece of coal. I tried so hard to shake them off of me with meditation and calmness as fear appeared; it had more than done its share, and it pressed on me to make my heart beat faster and hang heavier until it had full control. I consciously tried to toss fear away so that I could be the hard-won competitor against the fear that lived deep inside me. After a few minutes, they placed him on my chest, and he immediately stopped crying, bonding him to me within seconds. For both of my pregnancies, I pulled out an old Walkman and spoke words, formulas, ABCs, and other loving words to my babies. I think it worked, putting the earphones on my stomach. As soon as my voice was heard, it must have seemed familiar to him.

Over the partition came Joey wanting to hold the bundle in his arms for the very first time. It was then that I saw the most beautiful sight in the world, my son. I could tell by Joey's eyes that he was beaming and overcome with emotions that only a parent could identify with the moment a child has been brought into the world. "Biagio," I said. I peered into my son's big brown eyes and smiled at the baby, several times. He stared intently at me taking in everything there was to see. I was taken aback by how beautiful his coloring was; it was different, unusual; he was a very beautiful peach brown. It was like he had been in the sun. The color was more like that of a tan than the normal skin of a newborn baby. *You are beautiful, my sweet*, I thought, and then I said hello to him as he quietly took in his new world. He was a beautiful baby, a pretty baby, he looked like a little girl with delicate features and lovely wide-set eyes, but it is hard to tell with any baby when they are first born. *Hmmm*, I thought to myself, *I would have thought he would have looked more like a boy, but how can I really tell? This is dumb for me to think, and what do I know about how any newborns look?* Right about then, my OBGYN came around to the front of the drape to speak to me, telling me that there were issues with his genitalia and that she would be sending a urologist in to see me later that day. She asked if circumcision was an option we might be considering and mentioned we should speak to the urologist about that when he came to see the baby. With that, it was over; Biagio was here, and Joey and I were the proud parents of our very first son.

Later that day, the urologist made his way to my room to examine Biagio. After a thorough check, the diagnosis was a disheartening one, undescended testicles and a bent urethra that would need to be corrected in about a year with a surgical procedure. The news was disappointing, to say the least, Biagio's testicles could not be felt, and the doctor informed me they had not descended into the scrotum, so an ultrasound would have to be done to make sure they were in his abdomen. More frightening was dealing with the idea that surgery in such an area as the genitals was the last place I would have wanted for anyone to undergo, let alone a small baby. The doctor's instructions were not to circumcise the baby but, instead, wait the year out, and then have the procedure done, circumcising him when everything was over. I nodded my head yes as he spoke; however, the gravity of what he said hit home and fear crept up on me, coming to choke off my blood supply to the brain. I was in overload mode. Then, I watched him leave the room, moving on to get on with his life that continued at his normal pace with no interruptions while mine had seemingly been placed in slow motion. TIME had done this to me, slowing the reel to reel down to a snail's pace so that everything could be examined, turned over, pondered in the mind, and dwelled upon until there was no stone left unturned. Looking out of the window with my hand on my chin and a thick, heavy burden weighing down my heart, I gazed at the burnt orange pumpkin sun beginning to make its trek to the other side of the world. At that moment, I desperately wished I had my mom to cling to for support, but that was not to be. I thought about my mom and watched the sun burning hotly in the May sky. It's job? Keep the pace so it could make its way to foreign lands. Once there, it would wake up unsuspecting victims of the new day on the other side of the big blue marble. Was there someone else out there feeling down? A little sad? Mortified and confused right now? Or were there people out there jumping for joy this very moment at the good news *time* had brought to them? Did all of those people still have their moms for comfort and support when they needed it? Were they looking at the overripe pumpkin in the sky that was waiting to burst open and drip lava tears onto their faces? I was sure there were many people who needed someone or something to aid them in their rough journey. I truly believed that listening to a person tell their story, would blow you away. Everyone is carrying a burden, yet, no one wants to really know your secret.

When a pregnancy is announced in a family, excitement about what the gender will be, how the room will be decorated and hopes for a healthy baby are just some of the general ideas that circulate in our minds. Fleeting thoughts of the "What if's?" enter and exit our minds as fast as they can. The fear of jinxing or casting a hex or curse onto the tiny being growing inside a mother's womb is too much to ever consider. We don't like to think about those negative or harmful things. Rather, we push them down into the sinkholes of our minds, covering them with the silt and driftwood of old memories we like to believe we no longer need and bury. We like to believe that our children are going to be healthy and strong without any hurdles to leap once they arrive here on earth. No illness, no defect, no disorder, no congenital abnormality, just simply put, healthy. However, the idea that a baby is born perfectly formed, hewn from the Master's own hands, is more likely than not. When you stop to ponder the miracle of each child who is born without a physical or mental cross to bear, the thought of this is astounding that the miracle of life gets it right so many times.

News of Biagio's birth spread throughout our small town, and friends and family began to filter into the hospital to visit and see our new son later that same day. A girlfriend of mine came to see me and the baby and, during her brief visit, made a comment that gave me chills. After holding him for a few moments, she hesitantly said, "Kaye, I don't want to offend you in any way, but he isn't a handsome baby; he is a beautiful baby. He is the prettiest baby I have seen in a long time." I smiled at her and lay my head on the pillow. *Interesting,* I thought. *She sees it too!*

"No offense taken," I said to her, and after chatting for a brief moment, it was time to hold Biagio with some warm and wistful goodbyes. My girlfriend turned and left, and right behind her was Ruth and Joey making their entrance into the room.

You never know how strong you are until being strong is the only choice you have.

~unknown~

You gain strength, courage and confidence by every experience in which you really stop to look fear in the face . . . You must do the thing you think you cannot do.

~Eleanor Roosevelt~

10

The Five Bs of Baby Boys and Sometimes Six

Ruth was full of excitement at seeing her brother for the first time, and in her tiny two-year-old hands she clutched the beach bucket full of the five rules of a gift. The five Bs (and sometimes six) are bottles, binkies, booties, brushes, and a blanket as her gift for him (and sometimes barrettes). Buried deep in the bottom of the bucket was a small package of very girly pink barrettes. When I questioned how they got there, Joey whispered to me that she wanted one more thing for her welcome bucket, and so he obliged her. She informed me that Cake would want them for her hair one day. Cake, her imaginary sibling, the alter ego of infants that had manifested itself during my pregnancy in Ruth's mind had reappeared in the room today. As we discussed Cake, Ruth grew more and more upset that we would be naming the baby something else, and that Cake would not be the baby's name. Yet the nagging question of why she continually insisted that Cake was real had never fully gone away. As we talked about Cake, she grew angrier that the baby be named Cake. That dogging, creepy and crawly feeling wrapped its hand around my throat that time, sending chills down my spine all the while groping for those deep dark recesses of one's soul that had never been tapped nor brought to the light of day. So, to rid myself of my own demons, I wanted nothing to do with it…the idea of Cake. I brushed those feelings off of myself even though there were so many large red arrows hovering over the neon sign and an ominous picture being painted that made it too hard to ignore. Slowly, I ticked off, one by one, those bothersome issues off of the *something, some way,* and *some how* in my mind one by one:

Ruth's bizarre predictions and unusual gift choice.

The ultrasound technician's inability to be sure about what she was seeing in utero, my friend's commentary, and the words of our physicians:

A shy XY? echoed in my mind.

His penis looks a bit bent.

He looks like he's been partially circumcised.

Don't take offense, but he is not a handsome baby. He's beautiful.

Don't have him circumcised. Wait a year until we can fix the bent urethra.

Something was wrong, I just couldn't put my finger on it. That *something* lingered in the pit of my stomach. That *somehow* was how this all occurred, how it put a new life into the clutches of a lifelong burden. The *someway* was a lack of knowledge of how this came to be and what the chances were. That *is* the ancient vibrational field that hones in on all that is not in alignment with the universe and lurks deep down inside each and every one of us. It doesn't make a grand entrance, no. It allows time to linger casually in the recesses of the mind, awakening cellular remembrances of danger and fear. That primal awakening can make you sniff in the air in search of carrion or anything weak and helpless so that it can be done away with, removed from the thought, and removed from what it is that scares us most in our dreams. For this energy-sapping situation, I hunted it for myself to rid any negative energy from my body.

But soon, the baby and I would be coming home and I wanted to make sure everything was in order just like we had done for Ruth. I stuffed that *something* away again down the holes in my mind. I wanted to usher in the flurry of activities that would bring excitement to the household. I asked Joey if the announcement sign had arrived at home yet. He informed me that the "It's a Boy" sign had been put up in the front yard, and I was thrilled beyond belief because everything was in order and falling into place, or so it seemed. As we chatted and watched Ruth peek at her brother, the day seemed to escape us. It was truly a precious moment in time that has been frozen in my memory as one of the more peaceful gatherings we all shared in those brief hours after his birth. Biagio's feeding time came around, and Joey, using that as a cue to leave, took Ruth and left for home, as she needed tending to as well. We said our goodbyes, and I kissed Ruth all over, telling her I would be seeing her in a few short days as they walked out of my room waving goodbyes to me and Biagio.

They were headed to her grandmother's house for a few days to give her time with her grandchild. Then, focusing my attention on feeding the baby, I picked him up and attempted to nurse him. Try as I might, he would not latch on, and I noticed that although he seemed hungry, he was somehow distracted, somehow limp as if he were drained of energy. I put him back down in the bassinet and watched him for a while, and he didn't really move much at all. He lay there quietly with eyes drooping, quickly falling back to the place where he had been for most of the day, dreamland. But then out of sleep, he was awake and with a sudden lurch of his body, he vomited dark green bile all over the bassinet. I froze in place, my mouth hanging open in a gawking sort of way, not believing, or should I say, not wanting to believe what I had just seen. Realizing that bile plus newborn equals something wrong, I picked him up to nurse him again in the hopes that what I had just seen would not repeat itself. Then I ever so gently laid him down with a prayer that I would not upset his stomach. Then, bile! That is when the terror began to creep into my body from every joint and crevice within me, and the question of what to do next entered my forum of thought as a conversation with myself took place in the private arena of my mind. *Do I call the nurse, or is this just a passing thing? It's just a passing thing; will it go away? No, it won't; this is bad. He has been sleeping all day, more than a normal newborn does, don't you think? Yeah, way more than normal, and if you think about it, you haven't seen him interact. Let a few more hours pass and see what happens. No! Call a nurse now; something isn't right!*

Calling the nurse to come and take Biagio back to the nurses' station for observation took a lot out of me because something told me I wouldn't be seeing him again anytime soon. Sure enough, an hour later the nurse returned and told me that Biagio had been admitted to the Neonatal Intensive Care Unit, or NICU, because she had given him water to drink and once again bile was what came up from his tiny innards. My suspicions had been right; there was something wrong, and now my hope was that whatever was wrong wasn't too wrong. Instead, I hoped it was a minor blip on the radar that could be righted by a magic pill or wand that was magically waved over babies so they could go home with their mamas on check out day. I picked up the phone and called Joey, telling him what happened and that he needed to come back to the hospital as fast as he could.

Fear has a way of playing a tune on one's body by strumming each nerve ending and plucking away at the follicles of hair on our heads. It can even employ the use of construction tools such as a come-along to cinch tightly each muscle fiber of your body so that your jaws clench shut, making your teeth grind helplessly in your mouth. Fear seeps in like a cold, unwanted companion on a winter's night, petting the orbs of one's eyes as they shift aimlessly in their sockets for something solid to hold on to in their frenzied search for clarity. But this day, I felt like fear was beating its tribal drum in my brain, pounding out a war chant to warn me of its inevitable and eventual takeover. Every time I attempted to get up to go and see my baby, a headache would grow claws in my brain and take hold, scraping and slashing at the soft tissue making it feel as if it were going to swell in its shell. The pain was excruciating and would force me back into my bed on every attempt to get out of it. As soon as I lay down, the headache dissipated, and so, I would get up again and try to make it a little bit further. Eventually, I knew that wasn't going to be any better, so I fought off the urge to lie down and started my trek down to the NICU carrying the weight of my head on my weary shoulders. On this attempt, I made it to the elevator entrance before the drums rhythmic beating had raised to a crescendo in my head, forcing me to make a beeline for my room and my bed where there would be no headache when I lay down. For my next attempt, I figured I would get smart and beat the headache that was back in action. *This has to be from stress,* I thought, wondering why the pounding headache came at such a critical time. However, I was where I needed to be, and there was nothing that was going to stop me from seeing his precious face. I also wanted an update on the latest information they had about what might be ailing him, so getting inside and speaking with the nurses was of the utmost importance to me.

Once I learned all I needed to learn about going into the NICU and handwashing had taken place, I was able to walk through the doors and directly into the heart of the hive. There was so much going on and so much to see that every person in there looked like a worker bee tending to the precious baby bees they were in charge of. Watching the nurses buzz about and the machines click and hum, I imagined that this surely must be what takes place deep inside a beehive where the worker bees tend to the tiny little baby bees who need every nuance of assistance in order to grow up to be big and strong. Actually, taking in all there was to see in that room was overwhelming because between the noise of the machines, the movement of the nurses, the parents with their tiny babies, and the many different cribs and bassinets. I didn't know where to look first to find my own little one. Lined up against the wall was an assortment of different types of bassinets, some of which resembled glass slippers while others' glass boxes that looked more like aquariums than little comfortable sleeping receptacles that held the tiniest of children. Some bassinets had large holes cut into the sides with rubber gloves affixed to them so parents could reach in to touch and hold their infants without spreading harmful germs to them. Some babies were preemies, so tiny that I was shocked. Babies could actually *come* in that size? Others had obvious birth defects that needed correcting, and others, well, I'm not sure what the others were there doing hard time for.

Some babies had their parent or parents with them, others did not; some parents were crying, others were not. Some babies were sleeping soundly in their little glass slippers, others in their aquariums, while others slept in mechanical swings that rocked them back and forth at different speeds depending on how hard the swing had been cranked. Some rocked at warp speed, others more slowly as they came back in for a landing on Earth. They were scrunched up in tight swaddles, heads keeled over to the side with little knit beanies snugly jammed on their heads.

Those beanies signaled the sex of each baby, pink for a girl, blue for a boy. Curling ribbon which acted as a top knot fastener adorned the tops of these beanies which weren't caps or beanies to begin with but some large knit tubing that must come on a spool. In my imagination, Bertha the Beanie Snipper was at the helm cutting off sections as the sick ones were rolled in, her thick accent from abroad gaily shouting out, "Do you want the pink or blue? Which one do you want?!" And as the babies rolled by on their conveyor belts with inner tubes around their waists to keep them in sitting positions, a bathroom plunger would come down with beanie affixed to its underside, plunging the cap into place on each baby's head, ensuring it didn't come off during his or her stay at the Beehive Inn.

A lovely nurse came towards me asking who my child was; I told her, and she led the way to my glass slipper where Biagio slept soundly in his blue sleeper and knit cap. But when I got to him, I saw he now had an IV in his tiny arm which was taped down to a cushioned board and a cannula in his teeny nose. The sight was almost more than I could bear, and my heart sank like a stone seeing him like this. I inquired about the oxygen and was informed that his oxygen saturation levels were low. In other words, he was having a difficult time getting oxygen into his system which was mostly due to a severely congested nose. As much as they tried, she said, there was no amount of suctioning that would clear his sinuses, and oxygen was required at this time to assist him. I reached to pick up my child and hold him close, but the nurses kindly asked me not to as he had finally gotten to sleep after quite a rough time. I was upset over this, but I knew there was no way I could have stayed with him much longer anyway because my head felt as if it were swelling, and my eyes were bulging at the intense pain I was feeling. The longer I stood there, the worse my headache grew, and so, I left the NICU, telling the nurse I had a headache but would return later that evening to see Biagio.

By the time I made it back to my room and into the sweet, sweet bed, Joey and Ruth had arrived, and Joey wasted no time in making it down to the NICU to see his son. The news of the baby being admitted into the NICU was just as frightening to Joey as it was to me, and he wanted to speak with the nurses as well about what was happening to his son. Joey left to be with Biagio which left Ruth for me to entertain, so I had her climb into bed with me, and I hugged and kissed her while she began to look for her brother. Ruth brought her bucket back with her to the hospital and told me she brushed her hair nicely because she wanted to look pretty for the baby. Interestingly, she never really said *he* very much or used Biagio's name; instead, she would refer to him as, "the baby," Cake, or Brother. Ruth was having a hard time understanding where brother was, asking me if Cake went for a walk or was taking a bath. In her two-and-a-half-year-old mind, she could not comprehend him being there one moment and then be gone the next, so as to my best, I told her he had a bellyache, and the nurses took him to a special room where they could fix it for him. She asked me where the room was, and so, I turned off the television and did my best to explain. I told her that her brother was sick and, again, that he had a tummy ache, "You know, Ruth," I said, "like when you said baby has a boo-boo? Well, his boo-boo came out today, and he had to go to a special room to get his tummy ache fixed." She looked at me and said, "No, Mama, that's not the boo-boo; Cake have a big boo-boo." Her matter-of-fact statement sent chills coursing through my body and sent my insides into turmoil while my outside self was the picture-perfect model of a mother in control. If the truth serum lens was dropped down to reveal what my true image was at the moment, it would have not been how she was actually seeing me. Instead, it would have shown hair standing frazzled on end with soot marks smeared across my face. Every orifice in my head would be smoldering, smoke rising from each hole, curling and spiraling up, up, up to the ceiling and beyond with a mechanical "I'm okay" smile plastered on my face. Her words were like a gunshot reverberating through an alley, and my body reacted to them by recoiling from the meaning that those words could actually hold. *Just think positive,* I told myself. Not only was I nervous about Biagio's condition, but my head was killing me. I told Ruth that I had to lie down, so she scooted over and lay down beside me, curling up like messy cursive, and there we lay together, mother and daughter, sure of what she knew and happy to be alone with Mom again for a moment in time.

Shortly thereafter, Joey returned from the NICU with information telling me that the thought was that Biagio may have a meconium plug blocking his ability to have a bowel movement. With that news, I felt a wave of relief wash over me knowing that once he pooped, he would be on his way to recovery and out of the doors of the hospital for good. After that, there would be no looking back, only forward at the life ahead of all of us. During the rest of Joey's visit, I remained in a reclining position as I talked with him, and I felt terrific. There were no signs of a headache to be seen, and I was grateful that the mother of all headaches had finally subsided. With that issue behind me, I planned on going back down to the NICU to see my son once Joey and Ruth had left for the evening. That way, I could tuck him in for the night, let him hear his mother's voice to reassure him I was still there for him, and kiss him goodnight.

Once Joey and Ruth had gone, I immediately called for a chair so that I could head down to see Biagio in the NICU. Once there, I found he was awake, which was exciting; it meant that I could now hold and kiss my baby, but that excitement was short-lived because the headache had come roaring back with a vengeance, tearing into my head without mercy. Nevertheless, I wanted to spend a few moments with my son no matter how intense the pain was, so I sat in the rocking chair next to his bassinet preparing to pick him up. I would have to hold him gingerly as the tangle of wires and contraptions attached to him made it very difficult to maneuver and hold him. I struggled with him, the wires, and my headache, trying my best to keep my eyes open, but I couldn't. Every time I would open them, the pain would shoot through them, pounding my brain into a pulp. The pain in my head was simply too severe to even see out of my eyes. Clenching my eyes shut for a while to try and ease the pain away, I couldn't focus on holding Biagio. My head lolled and rolled as I did my best to deal with the pain and refocus on the baby I had come to see. Sitting there in pain, I heard a nurse snap at me nastily telling me that if I didn't wake up, she would take the baby away. Her words were a thousand bees stinging at me from all directions to do harm as if the queen bee was admonishing one of her workers. At that moment, I wanted to crawl into a hole somewhere in the dark and go to sleep. Instead, I mustered all my strength and explained that I was having severe headaches and couldn't see. Upon hearing this, she softened and began questioning me about how I gave birth. She asked if I had undergone a C-section and asked if the headache I was experiencing subsided when I lay down flat in the bed. Once she had enough information from me, she suggested there may be a spinal leak from the initial lumbar puncture where the anesthesia was administered for the C-section and said that it may need to be corrected. She took Biagio from me and suggested I go back to my room and lie down while she contacted my physician. After hours of lying flat in bed and watching the sun set behind one of the buildings of the expansive hospital, a physician came and met with me in my room.

After talking with me and asking me questions to assess the situation, he was sure there was a spinal leak and explained the procedure he could do to seal it. That leak or tear in what is called the dura, which is the membrane that surrounds the spinal cord, was causing spinal fluid to leak out which in turn caused the headaches. When I would lie flat, the fluid would then be distributed evenly in the spine, reaching the brain and making the headaches go away. He informed me that without the procedure the headaches could last up to three weeks. After hearing what the alternative was, I agreed to the procedure which he said would take place in a few hours, but in the meantime, he instructed me to continue to lie flat which meant trips to the NICU for the rest of the evening were out of the question.

TIME is like a machine, tick, tick, ticking away each second of our lives no matter if we are happy, distraught, facing a consequence of some sort or sad beyond our wildest imaginings. It lurks and hovers around us, fluttering its wings, waiting for the next event in our lives to be marked by it. Although we can't see it, we can feel it in the shadows, waiting. Why are we afraid of the dark? Because fear lurks there, or in a home, or in your heart and mind, telling you it's plan. One can always find fear lurking about, but between my extreme imagination and fearful childhood, it always managed to find me and welcomed me with open, bony arms.

About a half-hour later, my pediatrician's partner came to see me, explaining to me that there were new findings from tests that had been performed on Biagio earlier that day. She explained that an ultrasound revealed that there was an enlargement of his adrenal glands which signaled something may be amiss, or it could mean absolutely nothing at all. However, more tests would be run to ensure that he was healthy enough to take home in a few days. Tick, tick, ticking drove me almost to the brink of madness.

Almost immediately after her visit, the urologist I had been waiting for came to see me to talk to me about Biagio's urethra. At this point in the day, I was exhausted, confused, and wanted to sleep, go see my baby, sleep, take my baby home, sleep, and make this whole mess disappear. After talking for some time, he explained the basics of "Bent Urethra 101" and then informed me that this was something that could be corrected; however, in the meantime, I should not circumcise him; rather I should wait a year, come back to have the procedure done on Biagio, and circumcise him at that point in time. I was disappointed by the news that a baby so small would need surgery, but there was never any question about if I was going to follow the doctor's orders or not.

Mom always stressed following directions with everything, especially when it came to physicians. We were to pay attention to each and every word they said and always be sure to weigh the facts of whatever issue it was we were discussing with them or facing. When it came to medications, she was adamant about us knowing what the names of the prescribed medications that were in our charge, what those dosages were, and what they were prescribed for. Unbeknownst to me at the time was that Mom's personal prescription for paying attention would eventually come in handy.

After waiting for what seemed like an eternity, the procedure I had been waiting for had finally been completed, and I was on my way to the recovery room. I was excited, as tomorrow would bring a new day free of headaches, and I would be able to make the trip down to see my baby again. I couldn't help thinking about the fact that my baby was in the NICU, which made me have my own pity parties to appease myself yet wanting someone to fix it. He was there all alone without hearing his mother's voice or seeing her face.

In recovery, I was placed in a room with two beds in it. The room itself was divided down the middle by your standard hospital curtain with not much more privacy than needed to be had. It was your typical hospital set up, a large expansive room, and that oh so quasi-privacy that is supposed to be projected to the semi-room dweller by the illusion of the curtain that hangs between two beds.

While lying there thinking about tomorrow and seeing my new-born, I began to realize that events of an extreme measure were un-folding in the bed next to me behind the curtain. The realization crept over me like fingers of moonlight when dusk appeared on the horizon to bring fear. It was slow and invaded and percolated amidst my own thoughts before overtaking them and rising to the forefront of my mind. As I listened, I could make out the distinct sound of sobbing coming from behind the curtain. It was another woman, and she was not all alone, as I was in her space. From time to time, a moan would escape her and the words, "Oh God, please, please don't let this be happening to me," would come out of her mouth. Those utterances made me scared, my blood running cold in its veins and arteries upon hearing those words. What could have possibly happened to this woman to make so much sorrow invade every corner of our room? Tick, tick, tock.

A man appeared at the door of the recovery room and quickly disappeared behind the partition to her side of the room where soft mumbling drifted through the air, the words garbled as they reached me. I lay frozen in fear for her, afraid to move. Being in a state of frozen fear somehow reminded me of being afraid to breathe when I visited my mother in the hospital so long ago. I was afraid to rustle the sheets with my legs and took shallow breaths for fear it may poison her air more than it already had. Her pained cries were all I could make out, and they said to me she wanted out of this freeze-frame in time she was living through. *Someone,* I thought, *fast forward or rewind on the tape recorder of life, move the tape in either direction but someone hit a button in mercy… please!* Her pain was great, overpowering, dismantling every ounce of her being from its as-saulted scaffolding. She was in the midst of a nightmare in which she was wide awake. She was living a nightmare that couldn't be escaped from because her eyes were wide open and staring her hell in the face. It was a live loop feed from her own private purgatory that she would have to punch her way out of emotionally. TIME, her unwanted companion riding shotgun through the hellish dayscape of an incomprehensible reality, making her day and experience dragged out.

As fear for her began to mount in all my senses, more people began to appear at the doorway and disappear behind the partition. I assumed the elderly and slightly balding man wearing painter pants who appeared in the doorway first must be her father, and then shortly thereafter, a portly and somewhat disheveled woman appeared. She looked very sad; her eyes were red-rimmed and laden with dark circles and bags. *She must be sad girls mother,* I thought. Next, a man wearing blue jeans entered the room topped off with a dingy, white undershirt. He looked exhausted; obviously he was someone who worked hard as a laborer, perhaps toiling all day on a roof over hot tar not expecting to end his day this way. My heart went out to this pitiable procession of pathetic people as they marched sorrowfully by like ants attempting to escape an impending storm. As they passed me, I remembered the childhood song sung on the playground at Kimball Elementary School in San Diego so long ago. Only this time, I changed some of the words to match the somber tone of the moment. The ants go marching one by one hurrah, hurrah, the ants go marching one by one hurrah, hurrah, the ants go marching one by one, the little ones gone; he's left his mum, and they all go marching down, to the ground, to get out, of the pain, boom, boom, boom…

Sad girl's people hardly acknowledged my existence, and not that I expected them to; instead, they scurried past with heads bowed low, each of them carrying a solemn look upon their faces with mustiness and cigarette smoke stretching behind them like entrails that have been pulled from the carcass of an animal. It lingered for a while on my side of the room as if the odor itself wished to be the first to inform me of the open wounds suffered by the sorrowful procession.

As each person filed in, sorrow gained strength from them as time had served up its platter of deliverance to the room across the way. TIME had carved these folks up like bite-sized morsels for the taking, and there came sorrow who trotted in on her dark horse filling every crevice and void in the human cavity that was assailable. She made a grand entrance into the room as sorrow always did, wearing her heavy linens of pain weighed down by centuries of tears and keening. Sorrow needed no formal announcement in our room. For she sat high in her saddle atop her horse's back, dug her spurs into their cantering hearts, coaxing the beating life force into a gallop and casting her lasso out to drag over their human circulatory systems, gathering every nerve ending and muscle fiber into a tight noose. Yes, sorrow did anything and everything to create the heaviness associated with the grievous pain they were experiencing.

The more time that passed, the more sobs and tears were borne from that side of the room. Small, comforting words were offered, none of which seemed to be of any solace to Sad Girl, who continued to beg God for relief, asking Him continually why this had happened to her. Only I didn't know what *this* was. What I did know was that whatever the *this* was, it was terrible, because the entire group was overwhelmed with grief. A man clad in hospital scrubs appeared in the doorway, glanced at me, said a dutiful hello, and then passed beyond the great barrier reef of a curtain into the next room with Sad Girl and her family. Instantaneous silence fell about the room, and he introduced himself to them all as a doctor. He began talking gently to her, explaining that her baby was born with the umbilical cord wrapped around his neck and that if the baby survived the ordeal, he would not lead the life of a typical child. As soon as the poisonous effluvia of words escaped his mouth, a great wailing arose from that side of the room; the sobs were so loud they must have wracked her body like small seizures. Now she was Broken-Hearted Girl. I clearly felt her anguish because I, too, stunned and frightened by what I had just heard, wept silently for the loss of her son. The doctor stayed to give more information and answer any questions the family may have had, and then he was gone, shifting in and out of other rooms weightless as a vaporous ghost delivering news to those of us whose turn it was to hear it.

Wanting to give privacy to the family, I called the nurses' station and asked to be taken back to my room. There was not enough room in my mind to fathom the degree of agony that the family was experiencing. In my own heightened state of fear for my own son's health, bearing witness to someone else's terror overwhelmed me and churned every thought I had given birth to a coating of worry that covered me in a sticky mass of sweat. I needed to escape the room so that the air could clear for Broken Hearted Girl's family and prayers could find their way to their mark.

As I prayed for her and her child, I tried to calm myself by remembering that all the worry in the world will not add another hour to your life, but those worries just kept creeping up, so I continued to pray. I prayed for her family and for the doctor who had to deliver the news. I wondered what his weight must be night after night having to be the bearer of both good and bad news to families. How must the reaction of sheer terror wear on him? Did he have a family? Did he have children of his own that he thought about when he had to look a mother in the eye and tell her the child she carried for nine months wasn't going to make it? Did he see his own child's healthy and happy smile when he looked at a family and told them such dark and heinous news? Did it affect him only slightly because he had no children yet, or did it not affect him at all because he was still young and strong? Had time not worn his immortality shield down to a pulp yet? Had he given her some hope to face her fears?

What would become of Broken-Hearted Girl and her family tonight? Would she be okay? How would she get through this trying time in her life? When would her anguish subside? What about my baby? What about those enlarged adrenal glands? Why were they so big, and what did that mean? When were we going to get to go home? What about the surgery? How would I cope? How would my family cope?

I'm scared, Mom; I'm all alone sailing on the big blue sea without you to guide me. Why did you leave me? Broken-Hearted Girl has her mom; I have no one. I miss your arms around me and your hugs when I need them the most. Now. When I'm scared. And alone. Help me! Can you hear me?

"There is a wilderness we walk alone
However well-companioned"

~ **Stephen Vincent Ben'et** ~

11

Silence

B
ack in my own room, I lay there hopped up on worry, wondering what my little one was doing down in the NICU by himself. I had been instructed not to move for another two hours and so going to see him was still completely out of the question. I was a powerline strung high across my own bed, anxiety in my power plant supplying electricity that hummed through the power grid of my body as I stared at the ceiling wondering and waiting. Tick, tock, tick…

"Hello?!" the friendly voice said from out of nowhere. Turning my head, I looked to see another one of my pediatrician's partners coming in to see me at what I thought was a very late hour of the night. I loved this practice and all the doctors in it; they were *doctors* that we all wished to have. They were doctors that were made from special fabric and were cast by a special mold of physician. This practice employed the kind of doctor you only read about in books from a bygone era; they were always friendly and always there and always supportive, no matter what the hour. He wasn't one of the usual doctors in the practice I took Ruth to, but he was a well-respected physician in our community who had practiced for many years and had cared for many children in the past. Pulling up a chair beside my bed, he smiled and began by telling me why he was in my room so late. He said that he liked doing his rounds late at night because he found the hospital to be more peaceful at that time and that there were less interruptions which gave him more time with patients. With that, he began to talk to me about Biagio and the findings in such a gentle and caring way that I was able to release all my fears and worries upon him. My tears flowed freely, and he let them, never moving from his post and never pushing past any of my questions with scientific medical mumbo-jumbo. He sat there with me, human being to human being, and allowed the rawest form of my emotions to be exposed without lightly painting over them for the sake of professionalism. He calmed me by asking me a curious question. He asked me if I liked stories. I shook my head, thinking he was going to tell me something else about my son, but instead, he began to weave a tale about two friends of his who were travelers of the world. This story I will not elaborate on as it is not my story to tell, but it was the story of a couple who loved each other deeply. What I will say is that it was one of the most beautiful stories about the many different facets of love, living and dealing with the immediate circumstances that life can bring at any given time that anyone had ever shared with me. It truly showcased and highlighted the strength of the human spirit and triumphs over grief. After taking my mind in another direction, steeling me for the inevitable and relieving me of worries for the moment, the good doctor, my own personal Tusitala (Robert Louis Stevenson), sailed away, leaving me at peace. That name was given to Stevenson by the Samoan people because he was like a tribal storyteller. For now, I was not adrift at sea nor alone in the wilderness but on solid ground with a foothold on a little island of friendly people whose calmness carried me away from an otherwise grey and tumultuous sea of troubles.

> P.S., *Thanks bunches of millions for sending him, Mom...xoxoxoxo I miss you...and thanks for listening. I love you.*

Do not be afraid; our fate cannot be taken from us; it is a gift.

~**Dante Alighieri**~

12

A Revelation of Cake

Having been discharged from the hospital for a week, the C-section incision was healing, and I was feeling much better on a physical level. The blood patch had been successful and I was released from the hospital a day after the procedure had been done; and no more headaches to report.

However, on the emotional level, I wasn't doing so well; the fact that my newborn was still in the hospital NICU and not home with his family was unsettling and didn't sit well with any of us. It had been determined that Biagio would need to have a bowel movement before he came home to ensure his intestines were not twisted or kinked and that he could produce a stool before he was released. I couldn't believe it; I was actually excited and hopeful for shit to appear for the first time in my life. I also found myself calling the hospital every hour when I wasn't there hovering over his bassinet. Managing a toddler and a working husband with an infant in the NICU wasn't an easy task and with none of my sisters available or family relatives to watch Ruth for me; however, I was lucky enough to have Joey's family. I had to juggle the situation the best way I could. On the one hand, I got a few more precious moments with my Ruth, yet on the other hand, life felt empty and odd without my newest baby next to me. But, despite those bumps in the road, we managed the best we could to juggle the priority of the hospital around everything else that had to come second during that time in our lives.

For several more days, Joey and I dutifully traipsed back and forth to the hospital tending to Biagio, carting breast milk for his feedings, caring for Ruth, and managing the household needs as the stress of being spread thin began to wear on us. The only time we spent together as a family was at the supper table in the evenings, while the rest of the time we were immersed in caring for Biagio who was still in the NICU. Overnight, I would set my alarm at two-hour intervals so that I could wake and check in on my son who seemed to be, according to the nurses I spoke with, just fine. That news always worked for me; I suppose it may have been because it was late at night, and I wanted to hear nothing but good news when I was so tired and wanted to do nothing more but sleep away the madness in my life. But then when I went to see him in the hospital, I would notice quite the opposite from what they were telling me. Don't get me wrong, I would never mean to imply that those extremely knowledgeable and talented nurses didn't know what they were talking about; what I meant was that there was the mommy effect occurring in me. That sixth mom sense that tells you without a doubt that something isn't right with the cake batter. There was something very strange about his listlessness that disturbed me. Every time I was with him, he was sleeping, and no matter what position he was in, no matter how much he was handled and jostled, he would hardly open his eyes. When he did attempt to peer out of them and into the world, I could see it was a struggle to lift his little eyelids. I would rub his soft little head, kiss it, kiss his cheeks, rock him and sing to him, and the most I would get were fluttering lids with eyes rolled back in his head. Nothing would rouse him from his slumber. When I inquired with the nurses about his strange sleeping habits, they waved me off citing newborn sleepiness as the culprit. This lethargy worried me as I could not recall Ruth ever being this sluggish or difficult to wake up. Rather, she was an alert and perky baby, always gazing about as much as she could at this tender young age. This baby didn't do much; he just slept and slept and slept all of his time here on earth away.

Biagio was a big baby weighing in at nine pounds, nine ounces at birth, and so to see him wedged in his glass bassinet slipper next to preemies who were so little it was comical on many different levels. The nurses in the NICU dubbed him "Nunzio the Knee Breaker" because of his appearance. Biagio had what they called a perfect C-section head, round as a bowling ball, and it was big. Big like a small pumpkin big. I think that is where most of the nine pounds went, to his head, and because he was still so new, his little face was squished up like a mob boss calling out orders. All he needed was a cigar and double-breasted suit, and we would have all been in the underground baby beanie business. One particular day when visiting the NICU, I found him stuffed like an oversized turkey in the little swing they kept to lull babies to sleep. His head was keeled over to one side with the infamous blue beanie squeezed tightly atop his noggin. As I reached down to rescue him from his vice the nurses hollered at me in unison, "Don't wake him!" I was startled at the choir of voices and jumped about two feet back from the swing looking up like I had been caught robbing a bank. It was a comical scene at best, and laughter erupted in the NICU, breaking the tension in the air. The nurses quickly apologized and explained that they had an awful time getting him comfortable as he had been fussing for quite some time. Not wanting to disrupt the peacefulness of the nursery, I sat quietly beside him and watched him swing back and forth, forth and back, dreaming of where he had come from in his little time machine. Was he in pain or just uncomfortable? What was that *something* that I couldn't put my finger on about this new baby of mine? I did my best to shrug it off, hoping for the best outcome to everything as I sat listening to the swing's tick, tick, tock as it rocked back and forth like the rhythmic timekeeping of a clock winding down, down, down. I could only hope that tomorrow would bring better news.

After what felt like an eternity of visits to the hospital I found that yesterday's hopes had brought today's great news. Joey and I finally got a phone call that delivered the news we had been waiting to hear, Biagio would be coming home after a scheduled ultrasound today. Since he had pooped and seemed to be carrying his own, we were ready to rock and roll. A full week and a half had passed since Biagio's birth, and those days had been interspersed with a lot of tension and worries, so we were feeling as if we could now push all of those negative things behind us and move forward into open and sunny skies. Today was an exciting day as it symbolized the closing of one chapter and the opening of another in our lives.

It's really funny when you think of your life in terms of a novel; I personally wonder how many chapters I have had in my life. I am not sure of the number as the thought of my life being a book which contained chapters that didn't possess a profound effect on me until I was older and much wiser to the world. Now, at the ripe old age of thirty-something and coupled with the horrors of my childhood, I imagined I could write a series of stories. For my son, he wasn't even two weeks old and had already underwritten two chapters in his young life, the first one entitled *"Birth!"* and the second, *"Nunzio Navigates the NICU."* Perhaps his third chapter would be about how he escaped from the pain of the NICU, overcoming it by using it as a tool to be a stronger individual. But first, he would have to endure one more prodding by medical professionals before he could begin to outline and plot his great escape.

The ultrasound had been ordered several days ago to confirm that Biagio's undescended testicles were in his abdomen as was suspected, and it was the last thing that needed to be taken care of on the doctor's list of things to do for him. In the meantime, Joey and I decided we would drive to the hospital and stay with him until the ultrasound had been ordered before going home to gather up what we would need for the final trip away from the hospital. We were very excited that Biagio would be home by evening as there were many family and friends in the neighborhood who had waited patiently to see him, and now they would all finally get to celebrate his homecoming. As for Ruth, we left her with her grandmother to watch for a few days, giving us the time to settle in without worry for her.

All our neighbors had been so wonderfully supportive to us over the past few days, dropping by and leaving notes that inquired about the health of our newborn child. If they did catch us when we were home, they would stop over with food, and we would take a few minutes of chat time to catch up on the latest health news from the hospital, ask us how we were holding up and if there was anything we needed or they could do for us. They sat and asked so many questions about what was going on and why the baby wasn't home yet. Instead of idle talk, I explained what the NICU was like, how the staff members were good to us, and the questions went on and on. There seemed to be a true and genuine interest in our family's plight, regardless of the fact that we *were* the new people on the block. Our fate was turning into a gift with all these lovely people. We had a great group of neighbors there on our street, and their true concern, charity, and interest in us taught me about acts of kindness as benevolent humanness on multiple levels. The kindness that came from all of them was more than I could have ever imagined.

Today was the day to beat all days, and Joey was so excited, he could hardly contain himself. His son would finally be coming home where he could watch him grow into a fine young man with whom he would groom into a skilled carpenter just like himself. As Joey drove to the hospital, I leaned back in my seat and closed my eyes, picturing him as the proud father he was, walking with his son in his arms in the NICU, talking to him and making over him. Today belonged to all of us, but for Joey, it was a day of epic proportions.

Upon arriving at the hospital, I suggested to Joey that he be the first one to go in and see Biagio, which he readily took me up on with no hesitation. Joey always let me go in first to see our son, and today, I wanted to do the same for him. I hoped this would make Joey feel as happy as it made me to go in and see the baby as soon as we got to the hospital. I had been selfish about it; now I wanted to show some good will towards him.

After spending a good portion of an hour in the nursery with our son, Joey came out, and it was my turn to go in. However, when I went inside, it happened that my turn coincided with the ultrasound technicians coming in to work their mojo on Biagio. Always interested in what was being done to my son, I stood beside his bassinet holding his tiny hand so that I could quietly observe them as they worked.

The technicians wheeled their portable cart up to the side of the bassinet, pulled a screen around us for privacy, and began prepping for the ultrasound. The technicians were a team of two, one male and one female who, it seemed, traveled around the hospital bringing the portable machine to those who could not come to them. As she-tech began to set up her work area, he-tech left the room, leaving her to begin the procedure without him. As she started the procedure, an odd conversation took shape as the line of questioning she fired at me were not the usual ones you might encounter when undergoing an ultrasound. Those little noises we emit from our mouths that we call words carry power; they carry the tone, feelings, and emotions of the sender to the receiver, and her words were odd and disconcerting. Questions about the karyotype blood work flew about the room; those noisy sounds she made asked me whether they had come back yet and if I knew what the results of those were, blah, blah, blah. I began to grow more and more uncomfortable as her powerful words were encapsulated in the trouble that she knew about. And, knowing she was seeing something that I couldn't know or decipher by looking at her screen was unsettling, to say the least. Then, her partner walked back in. Tick, tick. He took one look at the ultrasound screen, and his head lurched forward as his jaw dropped open. I froze, feeling like I was going to pee my pants; his eyes opened really wide as he stared at the screen, and he turned and looked down at my baby lying there so innocently in the bassinet. Tick, tock. My eyes were bulging open; I could hear my heart beating, the blood coursing through my veins; *he*-tech looked at *she*-tech like he had just come face to face with the devil. *He*-tech was stunned. I was fucking scared. Tock, tock.

Blood was gushing, gushing, gushing, gushing at warp speed through my body, and I could smell the iron-ny smell of it in my nose. I felt like a racehorse at the starting gate, wild with wanting to know what they were seeing, nostrils flared, and eyes wild, mouth frothing, as I chomped at the bit. And so, I asked them in my coolest, calmest "I just smoked a whole fucking carton of cigarettes and chased them with a pint of honey" voice and looked at them in my coolest, calmest, "everything is fine on the exterior mask. "Are you seeing something interesting there, or are you not allowed to say?" Both, at the same time, chimed in together in a quick, Joe Friday "Just the facts, ma'am" sort of way, "We're not allowed to say!" And then it was over, and the ultrasound goo was wiped clean, and they scurried away with their ass cheeks pinched so tight they resembled rats attempting to find their way off a sinking ship. Something was wrong. I knew it; they knew it, and I know they knew I knew it too. As they left, they told me I would hear the results of the ultrasound from my physician and quickly beat a hasty retreat out of the door. Weighted down with worry, I kissed Biagio goodbye, told him I would see him in a little while and walked out of the NICU stiff legged and mechanically smiling at the nurses as they told me they were going to get the discharge papers in order.

The decision not to say anything to Joey about what had just happened was excruciating, but I didn't want to cause any unnecessary worry until I knew exactly what was wrong. Why allow two people to worry when one can carry the burden? I wanted to let him have the bliss of no worries if it turned out to be an unnecessary one.

The ride home from the hospital was a dreary one; it was raining, and the skies were ominous and threatening. I was already tired of waking to pump breast milk every two hours and calling the hospital checking in; therefore, my sleep was extremely minimal at that time. This birth experience has been quite different from the last, and I was glad it was coming to an end because I was exhausted. Between the C-section and all the events that had occurred after it, I was feeling a bit upbeat and happy that my son would be coming home on this day, bringing peace to my household. However, despite the upbeat feeling, there was an underlying feeling of impending doom hanging over me.

Once home, we sat for a moment, relaxing and talking about what we needed for the care and thinking about the last-minute details needed in preparation for Biagio's homecoming. This was a moment that was exciting, no, monumental, as far as I was concerned, and couldn't wait to return to the hospital to get him. Wanting to check and see if the discharge orders had been completed, I went to the phone to call the hospital and noticed we had messages. I decided to check the messages before making a phone call in anticipation of the hospital having already called to inform us that the orders were ready to go and that we could return to get Biagio. When I did check them, I didn't get the great news I was hoping for; instead, the messages were from five different physicians, one of them our own pediatrician urging us to call him as soon as we got home. Like in any good horror flick, the hairs on my arms and neck stood straight up, and shivers wiggled their way around my body just below the skin. What could possibly be the reason for their urgent calls? Knowing it had to do with something found on the ultrasound, I mentally reviewed the conversation held with the technician searching for undescended testes in Biagio's abdomen while my hand sat poised tentatively on the telephone receiver.

Has karyotyping come back yet?

Not yet.

Well, how long will we have to wait on this?

It shouldn't be too long.

Oh, okay.

Searching my brain for answers, I scanned my memory for anything that would give me clues to what the calls might be about. As I do so, I float off into the fantastical world of daydream land of the mind's eye.

I saw her running the handheld device over his tummy, me standing there looking to see with an untrained eye if I could make anything out...nothing. *Can't make out shit, damn! She*-tech's partner came and gave the whole fucking thing away with his reaction, mouth agape. He begins to catch shit eating flies in his hollow, hollow mouth with his hollow, hollow words. He spoke those echoed hollow, hollow threats that there was something dreadfully, dreadfully wrong. Those two monstrous twins begin chiming meaningless sentiments at me in attempts to throw me off the scent trail. One is ogling me with bulging fish-like eyes, the other wearing white, ghastly skin that was nearly void of color all the while staring at me as if he's seen something he has never seen before...so I asked again, taking a different tone in my mind. *Holy shit am I on the ride of my life?* I thought to myself. I feel anger rising in my gut, so I ask in my best, yet toned-down version of a gangster's impersonation, "So, ah, are you seeing anything interesting there, or are you not allowed to say?" My chin was up, and my mouth turned down; I attempted not to show *I WAS WORRIED.*

Oh, yeah, I think to myself with every cell in me not believing the tech twins. It was then that my vivid imagination kicked in, and I became a mobster. I took out my Ultrasound Tommy gun in my coolest mobster way for both of them lying to me in their coolest, coolest mobster *way*...with a stogie hanging from my mouth as I did it. Smoke curling from the end of the gun as they lay there covered with the ultrasound goo as I shot them down with it.

Having lifted my mood a bit and making myself chuckle, I snapped out of the detour my imagination took me on, keeping me from making a phone call, but fear gripped my soul, hand hurting from the death grip I had on the receiver which pulled me back again to the real world.

I'll call Dr. Williams, I thought; he was our trusted pediatrician, and the other doctors whom I called were only slightly familiar with us from the hospital NICU. I didn't know if many doctors were in their offices on a weekend waiting for a call from a patient's parent. Something very bad was wrong. Slowly, I began to push the buttons on the phone, each number making me closer to what I knew I didn't want to hear. Tick.

"Doctors answering service," said the voice on the other end of the phone call, and then after informing the answering service who I was and what I needed, Dr. Williams's familiar and kind voice was on the other end of the line. He greeted me in his usual polite and gentle way and then informed me that there were some concerns that had arisen with our baby. Tock. He wanted both of us to come to his office immediately where he would discuss the details with us. His words then chilled me, "Your baby is sick," his explosive words informed me of what I didn't want to hear nor what any parent wants to hear. As he released those grenades we call words loose, I was a mere shell of what I had been before he laid out the tripwire to make me explode from a step I was going to have to take. The words exploded in my mind, and my body grew weak from the work of the tripwire.

Words carry such mana or power with them. These tiny little vessels of information we use to communicate will slip so casually from our lips carrying the thoughts and intentions of the speaker. All the while not realizing that our words carry such power to the receiver. The essence and feelings we harbor deep inside our hearts and minds fly forth on the wind; each word we think, utter, whisper, or hurl at a person causes more damage than we realize. Words are deadly; they pick at the mind and bore holes in the spirit, damaging the inner self with the caustic cosmic "glop" those words are coated with. On the other hand, if these words are given with kindness and true care; they can nurture and heal the spirit of both the giver and receiver. The doctor's words were not harsh, but he carried with them signs of danger that my sixth sense deciphered and Ruth knew as strange. "Let me step outside," I managed, not wanting Ruth or Joey to see me faint dead away. I fumbled at the lock on the back-door with my fingers stiff with fear and stumbled out onto the back porch next to my prayer tree. Again, I repeated what he had said, "M-my baby is sick?"

"Yes."

"Sick as in could die?"

"Yes," he said.

"I need you and Joey to come down to the office and see me; I'll explain everything to you when you arrive, and you might want to find someone to watch Ruth as well." My heart sank low into the pit of my stomach, and I groped blindly for the door handle of my van so that I could open it and sit down. Consciousness spurred on by fear welled up inside me, and I hissed into the phone, "You tell me right now what is going on; I'm not waiting for another twenty minutes to find out what is going on with my baby!" I demanded the news to be told to me right then and there. I couldn't for the life of me imagine waiting to pin down a sitter and having to explain to them why I needed a last minute favor to navigate through my fear and keep it together for Ruth's sake, then drive the twenty minutes to his office. It wasn't going to happen that the meeting would be damn good and well near an hour away with all the things needing to be accomplished.

I sat down in my van, and he said, "Your baby is sick; they found a uterus." My head lurched forward, and my mouth gaped open with hollow, hollow sounds coming from a hollow, hollow mind and a hollow, hollow spirit. Tunnel vision set in; everything was close yet so far away. "Wha? I don't understand!?"

Between my sobs and the expletives I hurled at him with all the strength I could conjure up, I struggled to make sense of everything I knew nothing about. I was angry at him for telling me something that, at the moment, I had trouble comprehending, and in my stunned confusion, I asked him how I was going to tell this to Joey. Looking back over my shoulder at the door was a sight I will never forget. There was Joey in the window with Ruth sitting on his shoulders, both of them peering out at me in the rain, dripping wet, and muddy. Joey's face was stricken with horror, and Ruth's eyes were wide, curiously fearful as to what her mother was doing outside in the rain.

When any news that rocks the very core of your being is received, it takes time for your body to process it, recover from it, and then pull itself back together again. Then you have to talk yourself into forging ahead, then face and embrace what had been served up. For me, this seemed like a monumental task such as Sisyphus had. I asked myself how I was going to do this? I couldn't make my feet move, and I couldn't breathe. Rather, I was hyperventilating. With chest heaving and lungs contracting, I told the doctor we would be right there and made my way over to my prayer tree in the pouring rain looking for my God. "Why have you done this to me?" I questioned. "How could you have done this to me?" I demanded.

Have you ever squeezed a drop of dishwashing detergent into a bowl full of pepper floating in water? The pepper scatters like it is afraid to be near the soap, running for the border of the bowl like synchronized swimmers. That is how I felt, like a drop of detergent in a world full of people unlike myself. I felt surrounded by those people who have no issues, no problems, and at least one parent alive to call when they needed to. I was alone in a world full of people living lives that at the moment I felt I was not privy to.

The wet and rainy drive to the doctor's office lasted for what seemed like an eternity with us chugging down the road, moving towards our new lives in slow motion. With the color mostly drained out of my world, the view from my hollow, hollow sockets was skewed. The sepia-toned rain fell in rivulets down the windowpanes, and pendulously, my eyes swung back and forth, forth and back in my sunken face. I thought how strange and weird the world can be; in an instance of time, my heart had exploded, splattering my face with shock, fear, terror, sorrow, confusion, and guilt. Someone's prepackaged verbal utterances we call words had grown arms and logistical tactics of emotional dynamite were thrown into my gaping mouth; those primal heat seeking missiles had done their job well. They had blown my fucking head right off at the neck, rearranging my features from the inside out. As I cried from my playdough face, so did the eyes in the sky, mother nature seemed to be in harmonious union with her child.

The day could not have been a more perfect setting for the news; it was damp, dreary, rainy, and gray. It matched my mood and tone, which arose. There was a strange silence in the car as all three of us silently rode the streets of Hamden into New Haven down Whitney Avenue. Joey sat behind the steering wheel, rigidly staring straight ahead while I was twisted to the side, looking out the passenger's window to avoid eye contact or conversation with anyone in the car. Halfway there, a tiny voice chimed out from the backseat. "Mama, Jesus loves you," Ruth said. Ruth was the first one to speak on this heavy, heavy ride, and in her innocence and loving statement of faith, I felt like screaming out, "How could He love me? Just look at what He did!" But at that time, I didn't believe, but I wanted to in the worst way. She had unwavering faith in me? I was too jaded in my adult body. I wanted to believe that He did love me. Even though I knew He did, I felt as though He didn't, somewhere in the back of my mind. Even more so, I couldn't answer her. She didn't say anything else to me the rest of the way, but there seemed to be an unspoken understanding that those words needed to be said without any acknowledgment from anyone in the car. Questions were running full steam ahead in my mind, but the confusion of everything coupled with really heavy emotions made everything in the process a jumble. I couldn't make heads or tails out of what I was trying to think about. I was nervous and stomach sick about what I was going to hear from our doctor. But most of all, I was afraid. I couldn't talk or think straight and wished upon the most distant of stars that this would all go away. But it didn't, so instead, I attempted to focus on what I could, conversations I had with medical professionals and things I had overheard in the past. "His penis looks a bit bent." My original ultrasound technician, she also wasn't sure because the genitalia was questionable to her in utero. The conversation with my girlfriend drifted lazily back into my mind. *Kaye, he isn't a handsome baby; he's beautiful!* Yes! A girl! But what about Biagio? He didn't wake up; he couldn't just open his eyes. Period. His presence here on earth made him disappear. *It's just newborn sleepiness!* Not my son. I loved him, and I had loved him and still loved him with all my heart, even before he was born. Since they told me we were having a boy, I wanted him, wanted to hold him, and wanted to punch everyone away from him to make them stop saying those things about him and leave him alone. He was my son. That's it, my son! I walked, I thought, I dreamed the same exact thing over and over again. I saw him so that made him real. I kissed him so that made him mine. I hugged him so that made us bond. I held him so that made him belong not only to his new family but to me as well. After all, I had carried him. He had a little part in his hair, or at least what he had of it. He was going to like snails and go to bed with sand in his socks. As he grew older, he would get a high and tight like my brother Marines I lived and worked with so long ago. He was going to learn things from his father and carry on family traditions and the family name. My son. My son. My son and his little blue blanket, snug as a bug in a rug wrapped tight so he could fit into a glass slipper in the NICU while waiting to come home. *Will you be coming home?* From the fourth month of pregnancy and anticipating giving birth to a baby boy from the ultrasound that had been done, I had planned for him, prepared Ruth for him, and fell in love with him. He was only here for a moment in time, and now he had to vaporize into thin air right before my very eyes, condensation, exhale, steam, vapor, mist, vanished.

Arriving at the doctor's office, I felt my heart begin to pound away in my chest harder and harder the closer we got to the office door. I was Marie Antoinette going to my death at the guillotine; I only hoped the execution was quick and painless. I was frightened and the anticipation of hearing the news hung sick in the air about me having a child sick enough to die was paralyzing. The fear?, a rip of the unknown can render you unmovable and unable to function in the normal world. You become a part of a different plane of sorts, in another dimension that operates and still, the rest of the world functions strongly around you, oblivious to the fact that you are glued to the air that surrounds you. For me, the genital issues were a concern but came second to the larger picture of understanding how to keep my newborn alive and comprehending the complicated issue of genetics. The major shock was finding out that I no longer had a son whom I loved and accepting that he was really my daughter, all along having to reconcile that in my mind was something very hard to wrap my thoughts around.

There are many times in life I feel humans have experienced a rebirth of themselves. I often say, when I joined the Marine Corps, I was re-birthed by a male warfare culture which turned me into a different person than I was before. I was granted membership into that elite group of men and women. Now I was evolving through this, reverting through the creator's proving grounds of life that were turning out to be painfully constructive. This birthing canal was tight and dark, and there were no lights at the other end that I could see as of yet. I had just entered the thicket for the second time and knew not what life held. This mess of navigation would be blind until I reached the midway point where a pinprick of light would begin to appear. It was that restrictive feeling that each step takes place with trepidation. I stood fast, afraid of what life had to offer. Joey gently touched my shoulder and grabbed my waist, urging me forward. Holding Ruth on the other arm, he escorted us into the building and through the doctor's doors where Dr. Williams, the bearer of news, sat quietly waiting for us.

So as not to scare Ruth, Dr. Williams had Joey stay with her in the waiting room while he took me inside his office first to explain what had transpired. With great care, he informed me that our baby had an inherited disorder of the adrenal glands called Congenital Adrenal Hyperplasia, or CAH. The baby was twenty-one hydroxy-lase deficient, which is the most common form of this disorder, and this meant our baby was a severe salt waster who could not retain salt. Dr. Williams went on to explain that this mutation appeared on the short leg of chromosome number six and that the recessive gene had been inherited from both parents. In other words, both Joey and I had given our baby a recessive gene, one of which held her up as a special child that would need years for her to come to grips with. My baby could not survive without daily medications, one a salt-retaining hormone and another steroid to replace what couldn't be manufactured. He explained that, during the pregnancy, my baby had been exposed to what he called an androgen bath, causing the female genitals to continue to grow into what appeared to be a male. He went on to say that we all start out the same way and then, at some point during pregnancy, girls and boys begin to develop dif-ferently. In my baby's case, it was the energy in production from the adrenal glands that virilized her genitals so much that hers appeared to be male in form. All the internal female plumbing was there, tubes, ovaries, and a uterus, waiting to be discovered, and the blood-work finally confirmed it all. 46XX, meaning the baby was biologically, chromosomally a female. Then he pulled out the paperwork and showed me the test results in a cold hard black-and-white print-out. Our son was actually our daughter who would eventually be able to have children. That immediately raised the question of how she could have babies when there was no vaginal opening.

Dr. Williams informed me that, before she menstruated, surgery could be performed at an early age if we, her parents, decided this was the right avenue to take for her. He also stressed the importance of reading up on this condition and learning all we could about it, talking to parents who had opted for surgery and those who had not. If we were to do this research, we could make a well-informed decision. At this point, I was overwhelmed by the amount of information he had given me that confused me. I stammered through tears, "How do we know that Ruth is really a girl?" Dr. Williams shook his head and assured me that Ruth was a girl; there were no mistakes there, and he patiently waded through my questions until I was done. He also told me that the new baby would not be coming home from the hospital as medications would need to be regulated before the discharge date could be set. His advice was to go home and rest for the night instead of being at the hospital and allow the nurses to do what they needed to do to make the new baby better. Then it was Joey's turn to go alone, so I took over his watch in the waiting room, doing my best not to cry and keep Ruth entertained.

Eventually, we both ended up seated side-by-side in the exam room with Ruth playing quietly with toys that Dr. Williams had put in his office. The good doctor went over how to ease her into the revelation that her brother was really her sister. He coached us on how to tell her that the doctors made a mistake and told us that our new baby was a boy when she was really a girl all along. After spending a good amount of time with the doctor, we both felt slightly at ease with the information we had been given, yet we were so, so sad. Still needing to process the information given to us and work through the guilt, still questioning if it was something we had done wrong to cause our baby's illness welled up inside of us. We thanked the good doctor and left, making our way back home.

You know, guilt is a funny little creature bound up in a hunch by scars. Scars of women, men, and scars of all humans past mistakes and experiences. Those words that are unnerving never leave. Instead, they form fibrous keloids the higher the level of guilt in response to the guttural understanding of what we have done wrong. Those huge misshapen masses of excess baggage cling to us like bleach; it's a bottle full of our lives, carrying every ounce of our stinging record. They place bleach stains in our minds and bleach scars on our hearts if we had any wrongdoing in each keloid's process. No, they never leave; they lay in wait, incubating in our bowels like a dirty little vermin who hides in them, sneaking and peeking their heads out from behind the intestine they cling to. They wait to seize any opportunity they can to excavate their way into the open air of our thoughts to expose what we attempt to suppress.

Exhausted from information overload, shock, and the suppression of guilt, there wasn't much in the way of conversation happening in our home. I sat and held Ruth tight to my chest thinking of a new baby who needed me desperately. I wished the new baby were home with us to complete our family circle and make it whole. I wondered what the new baby was doing, so I put Ruth down for bed and went to the phone to call the hospital for a wellness check on our new baby. Identifying myself to the NICU nurse who answered the call, I heard her cup a hand over the phone and whisper something and identified me, "It's her, the mother, on the phone. Does she know? What do you want me to tell her?" That infuriated me, and the anger began to well up inside me.

"I know," I snapped, "I want to speak to my daughter's nurse please."

"Oh," said the voice on the other side of the phone, "just a moment please." New baby's nurse assured me that the new baby was doing well and would be fine throughout the night, asking me what time we would be arriving at the hospital in the morning as there were doctors that needed to talk to us about the new baby's condition. I assured her we would be there for doctor's rounds, finished our conversation, and hung up the phone. I felt assaulted from all angles, and that incident with the first nurse was enough to make me feel like I was being treated as the unabomber. Were they worried about my reaction to the news if I didn't know and they accidentally slipped before I had been properly informed? Did they think I was going to burst into the NICU with two breast pump bombs attached to my breasts with timers on them? Ready and poised on the *Jeopardy* clickers, waiting to send a shower of breast milk all over the NICU? I could see the headlines in the New Haven Register, "'Breast Milk' Bomber Strikes Again!" Where was the information highway at the hospital? Enough people had called me to deliver the news, so why wasn't anyone in the nursery informed that I had been let in on the secret so I wasn't treated like I had contracted the plague when I called? I told Joey about the reaction from the nurses, and he took the edge off my nerves by reasoning with me as I lay down with Ruth in the bedroom. I knew that everyone was ultimately looking out for my best interest, but when your mindset is all a kilter, nothing appears to be what it really is. A wise man once told me that your perception is your reality, and my reality during that time period in my life was warped deep in outer space.

I overheard Joey begin the arduous task of making phone calls to his family, breaking the news of the baby's condition through a river of tears. Hearing him in that state was more weight that I wanted to carry, *You've been so strong and supportive of me and in my state of mind.* Yet I was helpless to do the same for him. In reality, he had been my prime supporter, my reference point from which everything I needed to measure and weigh could begin from this journey. And there he sat in the dark, on the couch in our living room by himself, a shell of a man shattered into a thousand shards of glass, all alone. I stayed frozen in place, unable to help myself let alone unable to help him in the other room while his heart was beating buckets of pain. As he cried in the dark, so too did I, hating myself for not being able to go to him. But there was something in me that told me he needed that darkness to himself, he needed that space to himself, he needed his own family to talk to without me in it to listen, to touch him, to invade his hurt room, and so I left him. Not knowing what to do for him or for myself. Anger at my reaction in the situation once again welled up inside me, and realizing I needed to take control of something, I got out of bed and went outside to have a conversation with God.

Stepping out the back porch, I scanned the night sky for some sort of a sign of his existence. I'm not sure what I was looking for, but anything at that point would have brought me some understanding as to why this was happening in my life. After all, wasn't it him who said he had something he wanted me to do? Was having a sick child on his list of directions for me? Why? I thought I loved you and you loved me. Look what's done now. This is how you show your love?! I have already taken care of one person in my life here on earth, so wasn't that enough for you?! What have I done wrong to deserve this, and what has my child done wrong to have this appear into her life?! I hate you, and I don't believe in you anymore! And I realized that if I didn't believe in him, who was I talking to? Sheepishly, I ran back inside the house, afraid that if I didn't seek cover, he would send showers and meteors down upon my head at the vile words I had just ordered from my ungrateful mouth. Nevertheless, I didn't say I was sorry.

Once inside, I melted into bed and cried my eyes out. My mind began a journey of replaying every aspect of what had transpired and the many times Ruth had lain up on my stomach keenly listening to whatever it was she heard. I thought about that many times those words that she would say over and over that the baby had a boo-boo; the baby was not a boy but a girl that smelled like cake. Could she really have known that the baby I was carrying was a girl, and if so, how? Thinking about how this new baby had a whole life ahead laden with medicine, doctors, and blood work just like my mother made my heart break in two. I felt like I was in a wind tunnel being blown back into my childhood memories.

Why, you do not even know what will happen tomorrow. What is your life? You are a mist that appears for a little while and then vanishes.

~James 4:14 NIV~

13

Last Night in My Dreams

"Hearing bad news is never a good thing. All that was happening around me took me back to my mother's death.

"Mama passed away last night," my sister Bernadette tearfully told me on the phone. I repeatedly kept replaying the loop of what she had said and, in my pain, threw the phone across the room. Grabbing my throat, I fell backwards on the beanbag I was sitting on, screaming and crying at the feeling of the pain of what I had just heard. Those multi-tipped sharp-edged ninja stars I call words that I just heard from my sister hit me with precision and cut open my heart, soul, and the fear of her dying. It had all come true. "I'm getting ready to come out to help with arrangements, so hang on, okay? I won't be able to get there until tomorrow, so in the meantime, you need to call the hospital to arrange the pickup of Mom's personal effects and then contact the funeral home." Those words graduated from ninja stars to daisy chains swinging round and round across my heart. Then came the constriction that was tightening, tightening, around my neck, and I started clawing at my clothing as they began to restrict me, squeezing me tighter, tighter until I couldn't breathe. The thought of those things happening to me was frightening. Cleaning up so that you could prepare to bury your mother. The tighter the clothing became, the less I could see, breathe, think, hear, or exist. This was the first time in my life I had dealt with such blurred vision; this was also the first moment in my life as I knew it. The next pain came by realizing that the entire demographics of my teenage world had been turned upside down by being re-landscaped by the tectonic shift of the heart, felt by all motherless daughters. At the ripe age of seventeen, my beloved mother was dead.

Not being able to deal with her death well, I had a very difficult time sleeping. However, my mother came to me in a dream one early morning, haunting me by calling out my name. Her face spiraling towards me in the pitch black of quiet sleep, spinning, spinning, spinning, towards me in my dream the entire dreamscape was black, save for the tiny spinning disk that was just a pinprick at first. As it got closer, I could make out the recognizable features of a human face, and then I positively recognized it to be hers. As mother's face approached, I could see she appeared tired and drawn. Her spinning, spinning face had solid chocolate, chocolate eyes only with no pupils in them. Her eyes were glazed over and glassy. As well, the face stopped its death spin and stared at me with its cannula in place feeding the chalky, chalky face with its solid flow of oxygen. *"Let me go; take me off the machines now."* And at that very moment in time, I woke from my dream state and looked at the clock. Through magma tears that rolled hot and heavy down my cheeks, they carried everlasting paths and trails through my heart that would never go away. It was sometime after three in the morning that I had been spewing hot lava from my heart and out of my eyes in my sleep as the dream scared me so bad. Looking at the clock, the *time* read 3:30 A.M. Getting lost in the past, I once again replayed, blow by blow, the events that took place, only this time in a more detailed way.

That day, the phone started ringing, and every time I answered, Scripps Memorial Hospital would be on the other end.

"Who is your mother's next of kin?" the first voice asked.

"That would be my sister, Bernadette, why?"

" We are simply updating our records; where does she reside?"

" Tucson, Arizona."

"May I have that number please?"

"Sure, no problem, why?"

"Thank you, but I'll have to call you back, bye-bye." Click, buzz.

A half hour later, the second call came in with another nurse asking to speak to Bernadette. I gave her all the information she was asking for, and I asked, "Why the repeated phone calls?" This nurse stated that our mother had taken a turn for the worse and that she needed to reach my sister. She was as abrupt and quick to get off the phone with me as the first woman I spoke with. Growing increasingly fearful, I picked up the phone, and I called my sister in Arizona to ask if anyone had called her from the hospital and if she knew what was going on. She informed me that she had not been contacted but would call me back when she found out what all the inquiries were about. Ten minutes later, my sister called me back with the devastating news. "Mama has passed away."

Was that dream I had a coincidence? I don't believe so nor is there any written evidence that would debunk the experience that I had. Nor was there anyone who would ever be able to say anything to change my mind, for that matter. I believe that Mama came to say her goodbyes to me and ask me to accept her crossing over to the other side where she would no longer be trapped in the constraints of the human body she had given up for its soil-bound journey. I found peace in that thought because it was over for her, but I was frightened and all alone in dealing with her death at such a young age. With both sisters away, Bernadette in Arizona and Ramona in the Philippines, I was going to have to take care of a lot of arrangements myself until my sisters were able to get to California. I was devastated.

In 1984 there were no cell phones and household computers to put family and friends in touch with each other at the click of a button. Long-distance phone calls were still relatively expensive and calling overseas was completely out of the question. The only way to get in touch with Ramona, as Bernadette had instructed me to do, was to contact the Red Cross and allow them to do the footwork for me. What the organization would do in case of a stateside emergency was to put the service member's name on the base television channel ticker tape style across the bottom of the screen. There, the names of all service members who needed to be contacted within the news looped over and over again until someone saw the name and notified the person themselves. It could be hours, or days, before I heard from my sister which scared me even more.

"Why God?" I asked. "Why did you take my mama away? Why not someone else's instead of mine? Wasn't it enough that she was sick? Wasn't it in the understanding that we had nothing and now I have nothing?!?" From foster homes to state support to being dead-ass broke, this was the ending I didn't want to happen. I took care of Mama by myself for the last two years of her life, running and patching and serving and getting anything and everything she needed. This included pushing my childhood and teenage years aside for adult duties, graduation, and also chores. What was all the ballyhoo about childhood being the most wonderful time in a person's life, a time of innocence and a loving family? That was the biggest line of crap I had ever been fed because childhood was not at all special, fun, or memorable. In fact, it was downright frightening. So, who in their right mind would want to be a kid or bring kids into the world for this sort of life? I would never want to be a mother and end up scaring the hell out of my own child.

The very thing I dreaded had come true and Mama's prayer to live to see me graduate had been fulfilled. That is what she had asked for, and that is what she was granted. But, on the flip side of the coin, the bottom, just dropped out of my world, and I was all alone in it, swimming frantically to stay afloat. I never wanted to get married, and if I ever did decide to have children, which was a longshot since my opinion on childhood was a rip-off, my kids would never know their grandmother. All I knew at that moment in time was that I wanted my mama so desperately that I didn't want to be pulled towards that life. The very fiber of my being stretched so tight I thought it would snap off inside me leaving me incapable of ever being able to want again. Yet, there was nothing that all the want in the world could do to bring her back. How would I mature into an adult without her to guide me? Where would I go; where would I live; how would I support myself? I was an orphan in a world filled with those lucky bastards who still had the warmth of their mother's physical touch.

School for me during those last days of her life was a blur; my grades had plummeted, and not one school administrator offered to help me. I don't believe they knew just how serious my mother's illness was or that I was the sole caregiver in the home. Instead, I slipped through the cracks becoming the kid whose grades plummeted and who came from the other side of town, so I got displaced and misplaced in the shuffle of life which to me was really no surprise. No guidance counselor counseled me; no one asked me about my home life and what I was having to do for my mom day in and day out. Nope, I was a throwaway that was a little more than litter on the curbside of life.

Although my life seemed to not amount to or matter much to those outside of the house, each of us within the house had important rules to fulfill. Towards the end of Mama's life, there was only me left to make the household work, so Mama always made sure that every task was assigned, and attention to detail was the number one rule. With medication, extra attention was paid and there were times when she would send Bernadette and me out to the pharmacy for her pills, if Bernadette was visiting. Both of us knew exactly what she was prescribed and what those prescriptions were. Nothing missed our eyes or our fingers as we repeated the meds list to her. But once Bernadette was out of the house and back at home, those important tasks fell solely on me again. I was good at it because I had to be, and I attended all of Mama's doctor's appointments when she could still walk so that I knew everything about everything when it came to her. I was also designated oxygen technician by Mama, so that she could be hands-free to move about as if she didn't have oxygen-binding her down at all. Having oxygen during this era meant carting around a heavy, metal olive green canister that had to be wheeled around in a little two-wheeled white hubcapped, dolly-type contraption with a handle. On the top of the canister was a gauge which allowed you to control the flow of oxygen through clear plastic tubing that you placed over your ears and into your nose would deliver the vital oxygen to the user. Dial-up too much oxygen and the user was pie-eyed and Johnny Walker Black drunk. Dial-up a lesser amount and they either got their usual dose or didn't get enough vital oxygen to make them get up off the couch. The plastic tubing would have to be connected from the patient to the canister, and then the canister would have to be hoisted into place, by me, of course, and then guided into a circular metal ring attached to the dolly so it wouldn't fall out. Then the patient could take back the contraption by the handle and maneuver his or her oxygen around with them wherever they needed to go they were free. However, using this portable oxygen carrier was a little awkward as the wheels were fixed in place so that maneuvering it required some skills. During the early '80s, handicap ramps were still being installed, so not every place was equipped for those who needed special access, meaning, I, the oxygen tank technician, would have to heave the tank upstairs to improve wherever else Mama decided to go. She would strut around with that cannula in her nose, head held high, arms swinging and bottom shaking like there was nothing the matter, and I would tagalong behind Mama like a dog. I would weave and dodge people as she walked like she had nothing attached to her. If I wasn't right in step or fell behind because the tank on wheels didn't maneuver as well as she did with her best strides, the oxygen tube got pulled tight. When this would happen, I would freeze in place with fear, hearing and seeing the Batman words and sound flashes across my mind, "Pow, Bam, Splat!" This taut or tightness by the tubing caused the cannula to bend her nose out of place and ears to bend down which, in turn, made her glasses all askew on her face. Each embarrassing effect of the plastic tubing catastrophe would lead into the next one at warped speed, and it became a hilarious turn of events for me. She could no longer look cute with her face telescoping down like a piece of ruffled paper, and I, the dog girl of South East San Diego, got a sliver of satisfaction before I got my ass chewed. Even though I was pissing my pants with laughter inside, I caught holy Batman hell for not keeping up with her. I always hated that because the berating would inevitably be a public scene, embarrassing me, the lowly servant dog. I was in front of everyone within earshot for me not doing my job as expected. I think Mama thought people would be on her side because she was the sick one, and I was the ungrateful child who wasn't doing what I was told. In her last days, when she could no longer walk very far, I did everything for my mother, including cleaning up bowel movements she had on the floor, unable to make it to the restroom in time. Her bowels would let loose on the floor, flying like a home run hit out of the ballpark from underneath her long dress. I despised those moments, dreading the fact that I would have to pick up shit off the floor with my bare hands, nothing separating me from it but flimsy paper towels. The sickening warmth of it squishing under the towels and the moisture seeping through them would get to my stomach then through my nose. The noxious smell would hit my nose, making me dry heave as I scooped it up and carried it to the toilet. All the while, there still was Mama on the sidelines of the pickup shit event like some twisted bystander on a walker with a half-baked "I'm sorry" look on her face. I never really was sure if I bought her "I'm sorry" look. There were plenty of times I thought that the apology was conjured up to make me think she was sorry when she had really crapped on the floor to show me how sick she was and to make me have to do much, much more for her. I have those feelings because each time she let it go, she was in the bathroom doorway on her walker, not in front of the crapper, not in front of the television set attempting to make it to the bathroom but always never making it. She would let loose in the hallway right in front of the bathroom. Inevitably, it happened every time I was sitting on the couch where I could get a front row view of the shit ball hitting the floor at top speed. Then puppy dog eyes, and me, fucking ballistic internal anger rising like a red tide in an off-season algae bloom. I would scream and cry yelling how much I hated her as I played pick up shit; I cried, crying even more for saying such hateful things because I made her cry.

Sadly, I was too young to realize the power of asking forgiveness, and I never got the opportunity to tell her I was sorry for saying such nasty things to her; I believe it was because of shame. As much as I despised my role as caregiver to her and her being sick, I still loved her intensely. After all, she was still my mother no matter the physically ill wrapping she came packaged in.

Now I found myself driving to the funeral parlor alone, having to make arrangements to bury her on this last leg of her journey here on earth. At the funeral parlor, I met with the director who took me down into the basement where the caskets were kept. The stairs went on their way down, down, down, down, down to the ground, to get out, of the pain, boom, boom, boom; I had to find the right casket for my mother to be laid to rest in. This was my last task for her, and it had to be done right. I wanted something that represented our faith and my mother's devotion to it. Her favorite symbol of faith were the praying hands, and when I saw the casket with the praying hands in relief on each of the four corners of the casket, I knew that would be the one to lay her to rest in. I pointed to it, and the funeral director was looking towards it with his eyebrow raised, asking if I was sure. I nodded, and it was a done deal; Mama would be buried surrounded by those praying hands that meant so much to her.

Upstairs, the director went over the details of what needed to be done for the funeral, and I handed over the lavender-colored skirt and blouse for my mother's burial. This was the outfit my mama told me she wanted to be buried in on one of our evening chats. One night she summoned me to her bedside, had me open her closet, and pull out the lovely lavender set so that she could be sure I knew which outfit she was talking about. That is one of my most painful memories of Mama. Needing to bury her. Telling me what she wanted me to bury her in and both of us handling it, looking at it and telling her I would ensure it got to the funeral home is forever burned into my memory. Then that day, there I was, handing it over to the man who would dress her for the very last time. He gently pushed the papers in front of me for my signature, explaining to me that they were papers needed for her embalming. I signed them, numb to everything going on around me, and then I left, making the drive to the hospital to pick up Mama's personal effects.

Once there, I was given the very standard and personal white plastic hospital bag with hard plastic handles on them that contained my mother's personal belongings. I clutched the bag tightly, wrapping my arms around it and squeezing it to my chest. I pretended it was her, and I greeted her once again. It was all that was left of her, and it was then that I finally wept harder than I had in the last twenty-four hours because it wasn't her warm self but, instead, a cold plastic bag. This was it; it was final. No more macabre greetings from hospital doors, no more picking my way around spirits because the angel of death had finally come for her. It was done; I was done. I was now free of dodging death as he had already found his way to my mother's room and taken her away on his boat that floated in the air to pass by visitors so no one would even know he existed.

I finished the deeds in the best way I knew how. From the cold and sterile walls at the hospital, I had to make my way back to my empty house to wait for Bernadette, hoping against hope that I would see Mama sitting in her wheelchair when I got there. Maybe she would even try to make it to the bathroom and shit on the floor in the doorway; hell, I wouldn't even give a crap that I had to pick it up.

Waiting, I sifted through my many thoughts and the items in my mom's bag. And in it were her reading glasses, her wallet, a bathrobe, and the clothing she had on the last time. The very last time she was admitted to the hospital. I smelled her clothing and each item of hers as I lay on the couch with everything surrounding me hoping just to have her there, but nothing happened but silence.

All around me; the only noise I could make out was my pain and sorrowful cries rising up from my home on the couch. No television, no marking in the TV Guide so one knew when something was coming on, no more conversation. Suddenly, I was scared to be alone in the big wide ocean of life in my little bitty boat all alone, drifting aimlessly in a sea of nowhere to go. Where would I go tomorrow? Mama's life and all of ours are nothing but vapors, gone in no time at all.

"What is coming is better than what is gone."

~Arabic Proverb~

14

JESUS ON THE CURB

Moving forward to what my issues were now, I had not called my family yet, but I wasn't quite ready to make that call. I had more thinking to do about all of the events that had transpired over the last few days and sort through my own feelings and emotions before I could call anyone on my side of the family. Not that there were many people to call and not that I was taking issue with calling them. There was really only my two sisters to call, but I simply wasn't able to talk about it just yet right then. I needed to rest and have some relaxation so that I could start tomorrow fresh, ready to deal with the new mountain of information that I was sure waited for me at the hospital.

Once again, I didn't sleep well at night, and after tossing and turning in my own sea of confusion, I got up before sunrise and began waking everyone to get them moving and on their way. I was anxious to get started with my day. I needed to plot out how I would progress through it. Each step was a heavy one, so if I had some sort of plan of action, perhaps it would make the day a bit easier to get through. I had breast milk stored in bottles that needed to come with me, plenty of things to keep Ruth busy and entertained, plenty of items to keep me entertained in between shifts at the NICU, and the few religious items I wanted to place in her bassinet. Now that my checklist was complete, I wanted to go get my baby as soon as I could, but no one in the house was moving as fast as I wanted them to. I occupied space and time by pretending to make believe Ruth had needs while Joey helped finish up with a few last minute details, and then we were off to the hospital for the first time to see the new baby in her new baby self; what a strange thought process.

Arriving at Yale Children's Hospital entrance, it was decided that Joey would drop me off as feeding time was drawing near. Joey and Ruth would then go and secure parking in the garage and join up with me as soon as they could. So, wanting to get to new baby as soon as I could, I hopped out of our car and walked into the hospital to see new baby as fast as my legs could carry me. This time, seeing what laid behind those doors was the new unknown and extremely fragile children. I wanted Joey by my side as I went in, but once again, I found myself alone and facing fears I didn't want to stand up for alone. Reaching out, I pressed the button signaling that there was someone who wanted to gain access to the room, and the doors swung slowly open. There, across the room, was new baby dressed in all white. *White*? I thought. *Why white? What happened to his blue blanket? I bought that for him! Whose clothes is he in, I mean, is she in?* I walked slowly over to the bassinet; noises came from all directions, buzzing and clicking around, speaking to me with those deer in headlights gazes and frozen, frozen smiles plastered all over their plastic, plastic faces. All while they tried to assess how I was feeling and how I was going to react to what I was seeing. I took a deep breath and looked down on my new baby in order not to show any signs of anxiety. I wouldn't let anyone see one ounce of pain ripping the flesh off of my heart, right down to the steel girders that supported it. In my mind, I could hear the screeching sound of metal on metal. Pain's metal fingernails made contact with my heart's steel girders, and sparks glinted and flew off of it as my mind attempted to grasp hold of the move from blue clothing to white. But, the exterior stucco of me remained cool, calm, and collected. I smiled like an old pro as I acknowledge the sugar plum fairy nurses clicking and buzzing away around me. And there she laid, a brand-new daughter all in white, only she was in Biagio's body. I saw Biagio and then tried to recognize him as my new daughter several *times* over. Back and forth I went in my mind, over and over again. This would take some *time* to recognize her and her only as I kept seeing my son there in the bassinet. It was only human to do so. I knew that the new baby was my little girl; however, in the space of gray matter, my brain war was being waged. One side, she was a girl, but on the other side that was shattered, guided me to what I was viewing. As I had gone through a rebirth of men in the Marine Corps, learning that my child was born with a congenital disorder, was a third birth for me. So had the new baby been rebirthed into who already existed and now she was in the guise of someone else. I bent down and kissed my new baby's face, struggling to avoid the IV that had been inserted into a vein on the forehead. New baby was drowsy but a bit more alert than last time; I could see the new baby, and that made her real. I picked up my new baby and kissed her and that made her mine. I sat down in the rocking chair to hug her, to bond all over again for the first time as a mother and daughter. I held her as tight as I could so that she knew she belonged to me. I looked at her, and she had a little part of the side on her head that I thought would be a natural way her beautiful hair would fall when she got older and how her hair would grow. I imagined she would like all sorts of bugs on long hikes in the woods while wearing pink feather boas if she should choose to do so. If not, then I would put curls and bows in her hair. If she was too much of a tomboy to go that far, I could dream about it. She would wear her long hair in a long braid or bun like my fellow women Marines that I loved and worked with so long ago. That is how it would be for my new baby. I just had to work my mind around everything slowly but surely, one step at a time.

I did not stay long after my bonding session as I knew Joey was anxious to get in to see new baby too. I put her down carefully in the bassinet and walked down the hallway to the waiting room in somewhat better spirits to tell him about what I saw. The waiting room was empty of other parents, and I looked at Joey who was white as a sheet. "What is it, Joey?" I asked.

He said, "You are not going to believe what Ruth just said to me when you got out of the car."

"What?"

"As soon as you walked by the pillar out in front of the entrance, Ruth started screaming at the top of her lungs."

"What did she say?" I asked, growing agitated at him for extending the story.

"She started screaming "Jesus, Jesus!" With her finger pointed at the curb she said, "Look, Daddy, look right there; there's the Holy Firit!" Ruth was too small to pronounce spirit, and so it became "firit" instead. "When I asked her what she was pointing at," said Joey, she pointed again to the pillar and started screaming, 'He's right there, Daddy, sitting on the curb; can't you see Him?' "Kaye," he said, there was no one there. She told me He was looking out for you and the baby. I asked her again what she was saying just to be sure I didn't misunderstand her, and she rubbed her eyes, closed them and paused for a second or two, like she was searching for something.

"Did she say she couldn't see anything else?" He gave me the shivers because he was trying his hardest to get me to see what she was saying, and you know what? I believed her.

I sat down, thinking about my overwhelming feelings of how I felt when we were all alone in dealing with this complicated condition. We were humans really, alone on this big blue ball in the middle of the vast darkness of the universe. Were we just cosmic travelers on a piece of space pollen that got dislodged from its weed in some distant galaxy? Have we really always been watched over by three space travelers of sorts that can't be seen in our physical realm? So, I quietly asked Jesus, *"Do you really know when I set and when I rise? Can you really perceive my thoughts from afar? Do you discern me going out and lying down; are you really familiar with all my ways? Are you one of us sitting here?*

At the hospital, in some lonely little town, on a lonely little day, did he send a beggar asking for a dollar because of them being out of work? *Have I ever entertained you or your angels? I want to say I'm sorry for the way I talked to you under the prayer tree that night and ask you for forgiveness. I love you, and thank you for watching over me. I really need it. All the time.*

Why, you do not even know what will happen tomorrow. What is your life? You're a mist that appears for a little while and then vanishes.

~ **James 4:14 NIV** ~

15

Very Special Congenital Adrenal Hyperplasia

Spending most of the morning taking turns going back and forth to the NICU, Joey and I realized it was going to be a busy day. We started by seeing new baby and getting out of the way of all the physicians who were making their rounds in the early morning hours. Then after those rounds were completed and we had seen and talked briefly to them, we were escorted to a small room up the hallway that led away from the NICU.

There were a few of these little rooms, each with names on them. This room had been donated by the parents of the little girl whose name graced the door. I wondered who she might have been and what her ailment was, what her parents had gone through and if they had felt the same fear and sorrow we had. We had been given a special invitation into the room that many parents don't get to enter. It was like being a plebe and the hazing that goes along with it. This was an exclusive club we were invited to join, except this was a club no one wanted a key to. This was the club of shattered imagery, the club of misfit toys, the Skull and Bones of sick children. Only this wasn't the ultra-elite secret society club people dream to be a part of, it was the ultra-life secret society club no one wanted membership to. This club charged a steep price. For membership required everything you didn't want to give. That requirement was illness or surgery or the death of a little one. The hazing rituals occurred at all hours of the day and night with mysterious phone calls summoning parents at all hours. Sometimes the assignment or news on the other end of the phone line was so horrifying, the howls of anguish could be heard across courtyards in neighborhoods and high-rises. Shuddering, I opened the door I had been shown to and stepped over the threshold, out of the world of the ordinary and into the world of secret society club.

Joey, Ruth, and I situated ourselves on a tiny couch which all of us squeezed into like oversized peas in a pod and waited for the very special doctor to come in and talk very special news with us. We didn't know who this very special doctor was, but according to our very special sources, he was a very special bigwig endocrinologist at this very special hospital. This very special doctor that knew all about the very special condition new baby had, could tell us all about this very special condition because he was a very special "*this*" condition endocrinologist. He would be in very shortly to answer all of our very special questions. We smiled nervously and sat quietly in our very special pea pod couch while waiting, waiting, waiting, for the very special doctor to show up in our very special room.

Tension was running thick, so thick you could cut it with a very special knife, and both of us were sweating beads of tears that were popping up one by one by one through our pores like weeds through gardening fabric. Then the door opened, and we saw that it wasn't just the very special doctor who had come to talk to us. This very special doctor had a very special entourage with him. *He must be pretty fucking important,* I thought as at least three other residents, one of them very pregnant, filed rigidly in behind him.

I wonder if they have sticks up their asses so that he can make them dance a jig whenever he needs them to, I assessed quietly, attempting to inject sarcastic humor into my own psyche because of the jitters. They all seemed robotic in attempts to be professional at such a serious time, and that I understood, but there are some doctors who have much better bedside manners than others. This group, try as they might, were as dry and sterile as popcorn farts on a dry and sterile popcorn fart day. *He's like a rock star physician,* I thought. *He's so damn big around here, he has to have doctors follow him around. Shit, where can I get a gig like that?!* Calmness, self-emerged amongst my terror, I supposed to keep the information reasonable to maintain, I needed to stem the flow of terror. My caustic wit was a nasty habit that formed after my mother's death and became sharpened and honed in the Marine Corps. It had a way of showing itself at the oddest of times. It had become my way of dealing with and avoiding what was painful and/or deflecting what conflict may be arising in my life.

I wondered why the kind doctor had so many people with him; were there parents who would attack a doctor who was in a room alone with distraught parents? Were they with him to learn how to break such devastating very special news to parents? And why would they allow a pregnant doctor into a room to tell parents about their newborn child's disorder or defect? I found that one thing to be a particularly disturbing and insensitive overlooked issue. It bothered me on a whole different level that I find hard to explain to this very day.

Looking back, in retrospect, it sounds ridiculous, but the state of mind at the time would not allow me to move past it, and even recalling the situation and putting it into words illicits those very special and same negative emotions on a much smaller level. It seems time has lessened the blow for me, yet they still existed.

I kept glancing at her stomach remembering when I was like that, blissfully unaware of what awaited me in the future. All I could think was that her unborn child was healthy, and she *knew it,* while mine was lying outside the doors of this very special room, sick. It simply wasn't fair, and I wished ugly things on her that I am sorry for today as she sat there staring back at me. I felt she should be making rounds and following a doctor in the healthy baby section of the hospital, not here where the club members were writhing wildly with their hair knotted and tangled and bones pierced through the cartilage of their noses. She was too well-kempt in her Dansko clogs and well-combed locks. With nails nicely painted and makeup on her face, she looked well-rested and grateful it wasn't her sitting on the pea pod couch. She wasn't welcome here. So, I secretly commanded her with all the energy I could conjure up without ceremony to leave the presence of those of us who had descended abruptly into primitive life. She didn't leave.

And so began a very special doctor's explanation of the new baby's rare genetic disorder, CAH, with the very pregnant doctor sitting right next to him. There were big pre-packaged cardboard cutouts we call words that rolled off his lips slicing through my brain, entering and exiting my brain like a cardboard machete within a second of time. *What did he call that again?* I thought. I could not get my brain to fire off signals to my hand to write down what he might be saying. Instead, I sat there stiff with a pencil poised, frightened, and sweaty while trying to appear as if I was handling all of the news well. I wasn't.

He introduced himself to us as a member of the Pediatric Endocrinology Department and stated that he was very familiar with this condition. He said it was not a disease but a disorder that our daughter had. He explained that our adrenal glands sit atop our kidneys and produce hormones that are vital to life. Our new

baby's very special adrenal glands were unable to produce cortisol and aldosterone, which made them overproduce androgens.
The new baby had received two recessive or mutated genes, one
from Joey and one from me. He described a square to us, asking
us to imagine a box divided into four even sections. The new baby
got the sections with two recessive genes causing her to inherit
the disorder.

Suddenly, the pregnant doctor makes attempts to get in on the
conversation and look important, too, so she scribbles away on a
paper drawing the Punnett square, unaware I knew what it was. I
asked, "You mean a Punnett square?" I say in my very special intel-
ligent voice. Very special doctor's eyebrows almost fly off his very
special forehead as he answers, "Why, yes! That's exactly what I'm
talking about!" The very special pregnant doctor almost dropped
an ovary as she sat back in her chair. "Yes! That's right!" She pro-
claimed in sheer disbelief, seemingly stunned that the primitive na-
tives in front of her knew such a word or concept.

Actually, the truth was, I had just had a biology class and
learned about it a few months earlier. I secretly got a moment of glee
and a quiet chuckle out of that thought and then was brought back
to reality.

But soon after I had come back to earth, I felt that little son of a
bitch guilt picking his way to the surface of my thoughts. Although
I had no control over selecting which section inside that Punnett
square she would inherit, at the moment of conception I felt I had
some hand in delivering that recessive gene to her. I was sure Joey
had guilt too, because I could see him in my peripheral vision and
noted he was wiping tears away from his eyes.

The very special doctor droned on and on in very special medical talk as my thoughts took me back to the day I was told what the
sex of my unborn child would be. "*A shy XY?*" The technician ques-

tioned. I was somewhat disappointed when I heard that because I wanted Ruth to have a brother; now I would be telling her she was going to become a big sister to a little sister.

"She had an androgen bath in utero which caused her genitals to virilize," said the very special doctor. I snapped back into real time as he went on and on about the condition using terminology and words too garbled and confusing for me to soak up at the moment. Coupled with the fact that there were four sets of eyes staring at me like I was a specimen growing in a Petri dish, there was so much information being thrown my way, it was almost too much for me to process at the moment. "The blood tests we performed came back; the karyotyping tells us female, 46XX."

They explained the condition as simply as they could, turning the arduous task of getting distraught parents to comprehend complicated medical mumbo jumbo into a crash course in "Glandular ABCs for Dipshits" was something I was grateful for. They told me that the master gland, the pituitary which resides in the brain, is the controller. It sends the message to the adrenal glands to produce cortisol. Since the new baby's adrenal glands were larger than they should have been in a newborn, they needed more concrete evidence to confirm their very special suspicions.

My brain began to wander again thinking about the pituitary gland sitting up in her penthouse apartment with her panoramic view of the world through very special eyes. With a cigarette dangling out of her mouth, she sat in her easy chair and leaned back against brain matter, game controller in hand, joystick under thumb poised to make her first move on the big screen. The game system is plugged in; electricity is flowing, and neurons and axons are prepared to send messages down Electric Avenue. She leans forward ready to send her orders down south to all her very special minions. She pushes the joystick, and all the little soldier glands respond, sending their messages back to her on the big screen, except one. "What the fuck?!" She snarls, ashes flying and smoke curling. *Pituniatary* is fucking pissed. "Someone is sleeping on the job again!" She punches the joystick, sending the order again, nothing. She stands hitting the side of the big screen with a closed fist causing flashes and sparks. "Maybe there's a glitch in the hookup; this system is so fucking new the owner doesn't even know how to work it yet!" Again, she sends the order, lighting up cigarette after cigarette after cigarette. Nothing. *Pituniatary* goes to her command center and punches in coordinates to find out who the culprit is. "Of course, it's that little son of a bitch, *Adrenaldo*. He's always trying to get away with something!" *Pituniaitary* sits down, reaching for her more powerful ceremonial, very special vice, Kava. This will bring her more powerful insight as to how to spur *Adrenaldo* into action, pulling his weight in the superstructure that is being constructed. She is the kahuna, the forewoman of hormone production, and this SOB needs to get off his ass and back to work.

What did he say? I thought, snapping back into real time. I must have been sitting there staring back at them nodding as my thoughts went somewhere else in time. It was hot in that little room, and I was claustrophobic, wanting desperately to get out and away from everyone and back to my precious baby. I kept drifting in and out of the conversation we were having with the very special doctor as he lost me on some points and held me captive on others. *Why are we all crammed up in here?*

Down south in the region where very special intuition and reaction percolated lived Adrenaldo, an important official in his own world, but sometimes, rarely, he turns out to be a lothario, at least that is how I conjured him up in my mind. He loved *Pituniatary*, but alas! She loved *Thyroidore*, knowing that he was a more popular and well-known gland in the world that began to work except aldrenaldo. He also lived just a stone's throw away; his plans were to move into a cozy spot under the Adam's apple tree after the host had made its own entrance into the world. *Adrenaldo,* on the other hand, really lived too far away, down in the neighborhood where it was more industrialized, where factories processed, filtered, and stored what the city disposed of to keep it clean and in working order.

Whaa? Shit, I have to pay attention! Snap out of it and listen! I had shut down by this point, my nerves so raw and on edge from crying and worrying that attention to detail at this point was almost out of the question. Instead, I started focusing on a very special doctor's very special way he talked. When he would finish his sentence, he would do so with a big smile on the end, almost like it was practiced so that he could look friendly even if he didn't feel like it. Not that this very special doctor wasn't terrific in every way imaginable, because he was, it was just that at the moment I could have focused on a gnat shitting gold nuggets out of its ass in the southeastern corner of the room instead of trying to process the information I didn't want to hear. I was tired from lack of sleep, recovering from a C-section and having a toddler to manage. I was weak and worn from shock, and on top of it all, I had no family by my side for support or assistance. If Mama were here, she would have had so much information for me it wouldn't be funny. How I hated being without her! I suppose all those ways I conjured silly things up, then snapped out of them making them disappear from my mind. Those were ways I coped with being without maternal or familial support and what was occurring in my own immediate family. And so, I sat and watched for very special doctor's smile to appear out from under very special doctor's very serious face, and every time he smiled at the end of a sentence, I began to automatically smile back. I could see Joey bowing with a strange smile on his face too. He was all red and wet with tears, and his teeth would become exposed as he leaned forward nodding and smiling in time, with the very special doctor. I suppose we wanted him to know we were listening and understood his very special words.

New baby was so virilized that she had everyone fooled. *Well,* I thought, *Mama always said no matter what you were to do or become in life, be the best at it!* I smiled a little smile to myself and thought, *You did it up right, baby girl.*

"She will need to take medication daily to maintain her health, those medications being a salt-retaining hormone and a steroid to replace what her adrenal glands do not make, cortisol, and suppress what they are overproducing, androgens. Your baby will need special care during illnesses, and the first six months of her life will be the most crucial to keeping her healthy. Flu, diarrhea, and vomiting or broken bones can be potentially deadly for her and—"

"What?!" I heard the sound of a needle being dragged across a thirty-three record on a turntable, and the hairs on my arms stood straight up. "Potentially deadly?" I said. Joey and I sat upright in our seats, fear choking us. I had thought that since everything had been caught and taken care of with medication that there were no more worries; I wasn't even aware, up until now, that there were other dangers we would need to worry about throughout her life. Very special doctor had said "potential," but I suppose it didn't hit me in this way. Then the questions started to fly.

"What about when she catches the flu?" I wanted him to go over that with me very carefully, and I started to write furiously on the paper I had in front of me.

"The flu can be dangerous for her as can be a fever, vomiting, diarrhea, and broken bones. In the case of any of these situations or illnesses taking place, you will need to give her an injection and get her to the hospital immediately. You will learn more about how to treat her in these types of events later. Right now, let's focus on any other questions you may have about the condition itself."— smile.

"What will her life be like?"

"Normal as could be."

"How often will she have to see an endocrinologist?"

"Very often during her first year of life, and then the visits will taper to every six months or so once the medication has been adjusted to her body's liking. You see, every child with this condition is different."—smile, smile back. "Every child is on a different dose of medication; it all depends on the kid and what his or her body needs."

"What about her genitals; what happens with that?"

"The external genitals can be corrected. We will put you in touch with a surgeon who will be able to answer more of those questions for you. What you are seeing is not a penis or scrotum but her female genitalia which has fused together. We all start out pretty much the same in utero. In girls, the growth stops, but boy's genitals continue to grow. Because of the androgen bath, her genitals continued to grow. She is a female through and through." smile. I smiled back and nodded my head while trying to look like I'm getting all of this.

"Will we learn how to give her medication and injection if we need to?"

"Yes."

"Can this happen again?" we asked, thinking of future pregnancies.

"Yes, it can again," as he explained. "Basically, you have a one in four chance of having another girl that is virilized. You won't have three more healthy babies and then the fourth one will have this condition. Every single time you conceive, the potential is there." We all briefly chuckled, and then he waited for more questions to come. Everyone stared at us, and the three of us stared back. I started to conjure Clint Eastwood as an uncomfortable silence fell over the room. The Good, The Bad and The Ugly played its tune. Then, in the back of my mind, I thought, as if there was a fourteen-eyed western gunfight about to take place over a little lady in a glass slipper, and all were waiting for the first person to draw.

"I don't believe I have any more questions at the moment," I piped up. "And I'm really hot and need some water." With that, the meeting was over, and Joey and I were left to sift through the mountains of information we had been fed, trying to come to our senses over digesting it.

I was so glad to be back in civilization again, breathing circulating air and gaining some sanity. Ruth had been asking to see her little brother, and now she was thoroughly excited to see her little sister. Joey and I had been telling her everything Dr. Williams had instructed us to tell her, and she seemed just fine with telling us she was happy to see her and when could they play together. Although, there were moments she did ask where Biagio went. I wasn't sure myself, so I told her Biagio wanted to go back to heaven, and he sent a sister in his place, and that was why the doctors had made a mistake. We asked the NICU nurses if the new baby could be brought to the window so that Ruth could make some tangible sense of what was going on and see the baby she had seen only once. As of yet, Ruth had not been allowed inside the NICU as she was too little and could potentially expose the fragile babies to harmful germs. However, our request was granted, and new baby was brought to the window at the front desk for Ruth to see. They held her up the best they could in the window in her little white blanket that was three sizes too big. With all the gadgetry attached to her, it was difficult for them to lift her very high, but the staff was wonderful about everything. They did everything they could to make this transition a smooth one for us, and Joey didn't miss a beat. He held Ruth up so that she could see *her* little sister for the very first time. Ruth leaned over and kissed her on the forehead, and then as quickly as she was there, the new baby sister was gone, whisked away to be cared for again. Joey and I decided this would be another good opportunity to talk to Ruth about her brother who was now her sister. We walked to the elevator in silence and looked out the window to the parking lot below. There was sadness that hung over the two of us so heavily that I wanted to go home and curl up under blankets like messy hair and not come out until a hundred years had passed. However, that couldn't happen, so we went down to the cafeteria for a change of scenery.

Sitting in the dining area at the hospital, we began our talk with Ruth.

"Ruth?"

"Yes, Mama?"

"Do you want me to tell you that funny story about the silly doctor who made a big mistake with your sister again?"

"Yeah, Mama, that's a silly story, silly doctors," she said with a giggle, and with that, we began to weave our story of how Biagio wasn't Biagio to our two and a half-year-old daughter once again.

Accept what IS, let go of what WAS, and have faith in what will be.

~unknown~

16

Goodbye Biagio, Hello Faith

The sense of urgency to rename our daughter and to gender reassign as soon as possible was a feat I felt I did not have the strength to go through. The paperwork was being held for us to make the whole transition easier on multiple levels. All the medical information for our insurance company needed to be notified of the changes as well as the information going out to the social security office. I was sure there was more paperwork the hospital needed to do that didn't require our signature, but the basics of it could have been very complicated had things not have gone as smoothly as they did. I have to say that it was the sensitivity, care, and attention to detail that Yale Hospital provided us with that reduced the number of headaches and anxiety that could have been ours alone to deal with. With an express desire to get all of the paperwork behind us, we kissed Faith goodbye and made the trip to the office where information would be changed before being sent out to the appropriate government agencies.

I had been to Yale New Haven Hospital on numerous occasions to visit sick friends and family and had never given a second thought to the sheer size of the hospital; however, this time I did.

When entering through its doors, one is greeted by the information desk and a hallway opens up into an atrium with a lovely fountain and seating area. That environment is quite peaceful, offering the visitor a place for reflection and solace. Next to the seating area was the cafeteria and gift shop and, around the corner from there, the chapel. In between the hospital and children's hospital sat an enormous Lego statue of "Dr." Babar tending to his little patient. Now that we had to visit so many offices and places within the hospital, it became quite apparent that this hospital was like catacombs with hallways and tunnels that seemed to go on forever.

We finally reached our destination, arriving with Ruth on Joey's shoulders because her little legs simply wouldn't keep up. A voice from somewhere inside the office told us to come in and have a seat, which we did. It was very quiet in that little office, and wherever the voice came from, I couldn't be sure because there was no one to be seen. There wasn't enough room in that office for a fly to buzz about in the corner of the room if it wanted to. *Who could work all day in an office this small?* I thought. *Evidently someone can, wherever they are.* We sat there in the office waiting for someone to appear, squeezed into our seats waiting for the presto change-o now you see—um, now you don't magic show to begin. Would the magician make her appearance by coming up through the desk appearing out of thin air with the quick change of paperwork in her hands? Or how about just plain materializing on top of it amidst a shower of glitter and flash paper? Now that would really be *something*. Perhaps they would appear from behind a giant, billowing cloud of smoke wearing a cape with our presto change-o paperwork already filled out. Nope, there was no dog and pony show here. The so-called magician wore gray slacks and a simple classy blouse instead of a black cape. She came out from behind a little door that was to the right of her little desk in her too little office with no pomp and circumstance, no top hat and no funny little moustache. She smiled at us and asked if we were there to fill out paperwork for Faith.

Her question brought me back to reality, back to where I didn't want to be and gave me such a sense of loss that I broke down and cried. I didn't think I was going to have such a hard time dealing with this aspect of the change, but as she sat down and held out the old paperwork that held the last bit of tangible evidence of Biagio's existence for us to see, it gripped me with an overwhelming sadness. I was once again struggling to let him go as I eyeballed the paper-work with wild buzzard eyes. I was sending him off into the un-known by himself; in reality, we were in attendance at his funeral where no one came to pay their respects but his parents and older sister. We sat forlornly at his graveside saying our goodbyes before we buried him forever. Maybe if I struck a match and lit the paper on fire, I could incinerate his memory from my mind, sending him curling upward with the smoke and ashes into heaven. Maybe if I ripped the paper into a million shards, I could scatter his essence into the many winds of the earth, sending him in so many different directions I could never piece him back together in my mind again. Maybe if I placed the paper in a bottle and tossed it in the sea, it would float its way to the far and deepest reaches of the unknown so that he couldn't be reached in the depths of my mind. Maybe if I dug a hole and buried it deep in the hands of the earth, Biagio would be able to take root in the fertile garden of my mind. But *where would he go* in our minds, and *what would he do* there, when this process was over? Would he sit idly by forever in a dark cobwebbed corner of our brains? Would we never utter his name again? Would he be forever forgotten and remembered in some ethereal way as the child who might have been; one who once existed only in the mind even though he was projected into the "physical" body that wasn't ever his? He was merely a ghost, a vapor, a mist, a breath, imagining, and a perception which was a reality for a brief moment of time. Because of this imagined reality, was he real somewhere else, like heaven? Did we conjure his spirit because we made him real through the power of our minds? Because we had loved him? Can love be that powerful? If so, would he always remember me as his mother? Would he look down upon me from his loft in heaven and would he forgive me for casting him away? I didn't want to let go of the little boy I had fallen in love with as I carried him for nine months and had fallen instantly in love with him when I laid eyes on him in the delivery room. But, at the same time, I wanted to run out of the room and hug my beautiful daughter whom I had fallen in love with. The daughter who had the strength of ten thousand men, the daughter whose fight to live was an epic battle and had made my love for her grow exponentially because of it. The daughter I had secretly carried for nine months was the best surprise I could have ever had. Then I would want to run away completely, back pedal, do something other than be in this situation, as it was all too much to process.

I was in anguish and pain, mentally crying out to Jesus, my mother, the Saints, someone walking by me, anyone who could hear my mental cries or would care to listen, really listen to me when I needed to be heard. No one heard; no one listened. They all let me writhe around in pain, anguish and hurt all over my clothing, under my skin, and in my heart until I reeked of it all. I was sure that the vapors of the mind and mist of each heartbeat were surely being released into some realm unseen to human eyes, the stench so bad the angels themselves must be retching from the odors.

Joey put his arm around me and helped me recover my dignity before the woman who had been waiting patiently began speaking softly and gently. She was so good at what she did, and I felt comforted by her voice and her instructions. She had obviously done this a million times before, for those of us parents newly initiated into the secret society club. She was an angel in disguise, I swear it.

"This is the information that is going to be changed," she said, holding up a piece of paper. "Here you are; would you like to see it?" I said yes and took it out of her hand, staring at it with my eyes shifting back and forth in their sockets like the strings that secure them to the skull had been snipped. I saw Biagio's name and sex typed on it. This was the information that the hospital would send out to the social security office to get your social security number assigned to you shortly after birth. *This woman is going to erase him,* I thought, and tears started streaming down my face. She offered me tissues and time to regroup, but I wanted to move on and get this over with as I was physically starting to hurt. "Would you please give me the first name of your child?"

"Faith," we both said together.

"Middle name, please?"

"Christi." I could hear her fingernails tapping on the keyboard, and the thought of this being the final stop in my twilight zone made me start to cry all over again. Joey hugged me tight, and I clutched the old paperwork to my chest. With every click of her nails on the keypads, Biagio slowly disappeared from the world.

Once the information had been changed, I folded up Biagio's paperwork and tucked it into my pocket. I would eventually put this piece of paper, all the blue clothing I had purchased, small mementos, and a blue rattle into a pretty hat box to keep safe for the future. I would never be able to get rid of it as it was a part of her. This was her history, her-story, and these were her things, the very first thing she ever was, ever possessed, or ever wore. I would keep them in order to show her all about the story of her beginning, her metamorphosis into this world when she became old enough to understand.

As we rode the elevator back up to the NICU floor I said to Joey, "Today I started out upbeat and positive, and I felt like I could conquer the world when I woke up this morning. But I was wrong. It looks as if the day has conquered me." Emotionally exhausted and daydreaming of sleep, I couldn't wait for my head to hit the pillow when this day was over.

Ode to a Celestial Child

You play among the crocus, on a new spring day
The air is as crisp and fresh as sheets hung out on a line to dry
Your steps are tentative, just like the fawn's first steps or first leaps
at her mother's side
And the sun entwined its luminous rays into your softly scented hair.
When you turn to look for comfort from me, I am there for you
Arms outstretched
Eyes piercing your thoughts
Heart one step ahead of any pain you may feel
I am here, I am here, I am you.

My eyes shift a thousand times squared in their sockets watching you
grow into the heat of summer
Now your legs are as long as a colt in the meadow,
Features as delicately and intricately arranged as Fibonacci's
numbers in nature
You are a flower firmly planted in the soil
Although you may sway in the stifling breezes
Your stem is straight and strong as an arrow
When you turn to look for advice from me, I am there for you,
Arms outstretched,
Eyes wearing a knowing and understanding gaze,
Heart that beats in unison with yours,
I am here, I am here, I am you.

My watch over you has relaxed as autumn descends upon me
You are like the mighty oak now
With roots that have stretched deep and wide

I marvel at your essence as it materializes,
then dances and plays on your lips in the crisp air
I feel the magic that life still holds for you
as you kiss my weathered cheek
And when you turn to ask my opinion, I am there for you
Arms welcoming your hug
Eyes grateful for the sight of you
Heart filled with love for you
I am here, I am here, I am you.

I keep vigil over you in my mind's eye now
Replaying the newness of you in spring
You are my crowning glory
My bouquet of beauty blankets me in blessings
My adornment of honor for a job well done too.
When you turn to be with me and I am no longer there,
Know in your memory my arms were always outstretched to you
My eyes will forever watch over you
My heart beats surreptitiously inside of yours
I *was* there, I *am* here, I **AM** you.

KC

"Those blessings are sweetest that are won with prayer and worn with thanks."

— **Thomas Goodwin~**

17

You Almost Missed Your Blessing

Evening finally came, and when I got home, I went directly to the shower where I stayed for about thirty minutes in the hot steam crying and praying, praying and crying. I was completely overwhelmed one minute; the next, I was okay with everything. I didn't know if I was coming or going and didn't know where to start or end. There were many times in my life that I had felt all alone, but this was one of those times that I could have been in a room full of people celebrating me. I would have still felt as if they couldn't have understood the depth or gravity of the situation I was attempting to compete with. Although I had Joey's family around me, they still weren't the family I had grown up with, fought with, been guided by as a child, and been loved as I grew into an adolescent. His mother wasn't *my* mother, and I wanted *my* mother, the one who gave birth to me, scolded me, pissed me off when she wouldn't let me do something I wanted to. Even though I knew she was right and couldn't give me an allowance like all the other kid's moms who did give them an allowance that I went to school with.

Underlying currents of negativity had been simmering hotly in our household as of late with phone calls to me and rumors circulating around town that were getting back to me about the birth of our child. There were things being said about me, and they weren't very kind. Joey had attempted to put everything to rest by handling it himself; in my opinion, he didn't do a good enough job for me. I know that sounds crass, but at the time it made perfect sense to me. I wanted him to ride in like a swashbuckling pirate and save me, the damsel in distress, by kicking ass and taking no prisoners. Slashing, dashing, and hurting people just as deeply as they had hurt my already deeply wounded heart. I had bigger fish to fry than to fight battles outside my home with people whose real intentions were not clear to me. Instead, I wanted Joey to be the buffer and protect me from them all. Those rumors had enraged and hurt me. I vowed to myself that no one's ignorant comments out of fear and the unknown would stand in the way of caring for my newborn daughter and the healing my own family needed to do.

I have to admit, although I overlooked the ugliness, I didn't avoid being pissed off about it. I didn't take a Stepford wife approach and smile nicely about the whole issue, no. I was a son of a bitch about it. But I stayed my distance and let the chips fall where they may, not confronting anyone about anything. Would I have liked to? You bet. Would I have gnawed on their jugulars like a rabid vampire if allowed? Most assuredly. But why not? Because I was too tired, too defeated, too engrossed in coping, learning, and dealing with the task at hand. In other words, I had bigger fish to fry than bottom feed and dwell in the muck with those of them that chose to voice their opinions without knowing what they were talking about. Instead, I was mystified that a close knit town could do nothing better than circle like sharks at a bloodbath waiting to take their own chunk out of my ass when I was already bleeding out instead of wholeheartedly being there to love me and support me unconditionally in such a time of need.

And with that I will say that there is no replacement in the world for your own mother, and when I say mother, I refer not necessarily to the one who gave birth to you as that does not apply to all of us in all circumstances, but the one who has loved or nurtured you unconditionally and has and will make everything that is wrong in the world right for you at the drop of a hat. I am referring to the mother who held your heart in her hands and kissed your tears away as you cried because your heart was broken for the very first time by the boy who ripped it out of your chest and stomped it on the ground. The mother who took care of you when you were sick by wiping your ass when you were too small to do it yourself. The mother who held your hair back when you vomited up the two pounds of zucchini bread loaded with butter she told you not to eat. Then, after doing all of that for you, the mother who went off to the kitchen to make you her world famous chicken noodle soup, never forgetting to add her most secret ingredient to the pot, love, so that your tummy would feel better. The mother who always loved you in your most beautiful and most awkward times in life and never saw you any different to her than you were, always…just…beautiful.

Life without my mother had been long and tough, and I missed her every single day of, but now, oh, but now I wished for her like I had never wished for anything else in the world. I wished for her so hard I felt like I could turn myself inside out from wishing so desperately. There were some of Joey's family members that were always there for us, but *my* sisters were far away, and I had no one from my own close family circle to draw their wagons around me in support, to protect me from prying eyes, and no one to clear the thicket with me. No one to sit with their arms around me as the doctors explained things, no one to hold my heart in their hands as I cried my eyes out. No one wanted to go out into the wild and do a proper and *correct* job of explaining to friends and neighbors our daughter's condition for me while I coped. No one would make me a special bowl of love so that my churning guts would feel better, no one. There was no one I trusted to do the job for me in the fashion I would expect it to be done in, no one except myself. Aside from Joey, I was the only person I had; that feeling was not a good one.

I was up and down through the night calling the hospital to get updates on Faith and to sort through the many thoughts in my mind. I love the night because, at night, there is silence, pure, sweet quiet that is uninterrupted. Within the night there is room for your thoughts to move about, unrestricted by the assaults of the day. It is a time when meditative thoughts and antiseptic prayers can flow freely to mend the open sores of the spirit and knit together the splintered and fractured pieces of your heart. As well, there are no phones ringing, no explaining that needs to be done, and no "well-meaning" people attempting to pump information from me before it is ready to be shared. Mostly, there were well-meaning friends and acquaintances telling me in all earnestness, "I could never handle that. God gives us what we can handle, Kaye; you are so strong, that's why he gave this to you! He knew *you* could handle it."

How I hated hearing those puss-infused pockets of infection we call words that were sent my way like airborne viruses. When I did hear them, a searing anger and hate would well up inside of me that wanted to burst out of my lips in a fury of metal I called words. I wanted to send them out to those who had infected me with their words, jabbing at them with the power of a prize fighter's fists. Instead, I would pretend to stand there weak and confused in my heartbreak and anger, looking at them through teary eyes, nodding my head yes and agreeing with their statement in the hopes they would just go away. But, instead, I would be thinking back to them,

Ah, that's why God gave you that bell pepper you wear as the nose on your face because He knew I could never handle that! No, there was nothing around except the plain, beautiful quiet in the middle of the silky night where you are free to hear yourself think without interruption from anyone or anything to bother you and your thoughts. The night envelopes you in its darkness, wraps its sultry arms around you, and seduces you with its isolation. It is like velvet being cloaked about you when you need it, and I loved the darkness when it came. I carefully stepped into the calmness of quietness the inky blackness brought with it. After a few hours of solace, I found myself getting drowsy and drifting off to sleep feeling much more at ease than I did all day long.

The next morning came fast with the rays of sunshine streaming through the windows in my bedroom. *It's time to rise and shine already,* I thought; time to go see my Faith. My heart was still very heavy, not at all upbeat and happy like it was the day before when I got up. Mood swings were something I was sure I would experience for a while, not to mention postpartum blues that might be mixed into the recipe as well. It was all I could do to raise myself out of bed, but I managed, swinging my heavy legs out and setting my anvil feet on the floor. I looked back over my shoulder at Ruth and Joey sleeping so peacefully and sighed, wishing that I could be sleeping too instead of sitting and feeling heavy. I asked God, *Why did You let this happen to me, and why won't You ANSWER?! Why have You left me alone to fend for myself through all of this?! I'm so damn mad!* Then it hit me like a bolt out of the blue. Like some mysterious delivery system existed in another realm, the message popped into my mind as clear as day. I heard the words being spoken in my mind, they weren't *my* words, but they were in *my* thoughts. Let me clarify what I mean here. The words weren't spoken to me by some disembodied booming voice that commanded me to listen. No, it was my voice, like what you would hear when you think of something like errands you have to run or what you are going to make or buy for dinner. But I *wasn't* thinking about them. It was as if I were eavesdropping on someone else's thoughts and hearing them in my head with my own familiar voice. What I heard made a light bulb click on in my brain.

You egocentric selfish human being! In the midst of your own groveling and whining, you failed to see the true blessing in all of this. You have not always walked a straight path. Despite all of your ill ways, I still found you worthy enough to care for such a precious soul! In my self-centeredness, I had been asking why this had happened to *me*, not anyone else, just me. In all my prayers and questioning if anyone was there hearing me, listening to me, carrying me through this I knew then that He was, He had been there the whole time supporting me through each task and burden in life. He had never left me; it was I who had abandoned Him in one of my darkest hours questioning His love for me.

I had received three precious things, Ruth, my steadfast and loving daughter, and two cherished gifts of Faith. One faith was given to me long ago in a dream that gave me the ability to believe in something on a deeper and more meaningful level. This faith allowed me to believe in myself and trust in the process of becoming a mother. This faith allowed me to experience what love really meant on different planes, and for that alone I could not be more thankful. The other was my daughter Faith who tested the first faith to see how strong it was, to prove how strong love can be. The tensile strength of those mother-child bonds could not be broken, no matter the issue, and because of her lesson given to me, I loved her more every day. For those gifts I am eternally grateful, and both my girls now needed and depended on me to be there for them. It was then I knew that the circle had become complete in receiving this blessing. Biagio could now rest in peace in my mind, allowing Faith to stake her claim in the world by announcing her arrival more loudly than most babies would ever have the chance to do.

At the hospital I drank in the beauty of her existence as I sat by her side and knew then that I had been blessed beyond measure. He knew exactly what He was doing by blessing us with this new daughter for every sorrowful step; He allowed time to be the consistent factor that delivered the gifts of renewed hope and faith. I thought about what my girlfriend said about my son being beautiful, and I smiled again. Faith's inner beauty had shone through like a beacon of light even when we did not know she was a girl. I again went over in my mind the phrase my mother used to say, *Whatever you do in life, I will always be proud of you, but make sure whatever it is that you do, you ensure you are the best at it.* Mother also used to say to be able to get through life's adversities, one must do so with their heads held high and faces turned upwards towards the sky. That fit my Faith; she entered the world with a bang and never looked back. Through her struggle for survival, she was born twice into the same fearfully and wonderfully made body that God had sent her here with. What a testament to life itself she was, and I was fortunate enough to be able to witness the Lord's works; and she was one of them.

Reflecting back on that first dream and the message that came with it about something there was for me to do made me ask myself if it was Ruth's birth or Faith's birth or both of their births I was to experience as a woman. Maybe the plan had nothing to do with me at all; perhaps I was just a vehicle or vessel to bring these children into the world for something else to occur later down the road. That something else didn't have to be great or epic in the standard way we see and view accomplishments and achievements on a grand scale, no. That isn't what is important in life. It is the small and seem-

ingly insignificant things that we do for one another that are significant and can compound into profound moments in a person's life.

Today, a small deed was being done for a very small person who
deserved her day in the sun just like any other deserving individual.
Joey had gone home to meet the sign company at our house. They
were coming to change the "It's a Boy!" sign to an "It's a Girl!" Faith,
nine pounds, nine ounces. The sign company had been very empa-
thetic to our needs and was more than willing to return and take
down the old sign and replace it with Faith's information. The day
we named her, Joey had turned to me and said, "She's going to have
her day, Kaye, just like Ruth did; Faith gets her day too!" Then he
left with Ruth to give Faith her day in the sun.

Sitting with Faith I was able to take her in and see the little girl
she would develop into and grow before my eyes. There were still
times I would catch fleeting glances of Biagio, but Faith would
quickly come back into view. Biagio was losing his grasp on reality,
and Faith was gaining her solid foothold in my perception. There
were still tearful moments of pain that would well up from time to
time, and although this particular life lesson had been a baptism
by fire, I now had a different set of glasses on my face with lenses
that showed me the world in a far different light than I had ever
viewed it in before. Instead of being in the world and looking
through foggy lenses, I felt like this life-altering experience moved
me away from that, giving me a room with a much clearer view so
that I could now look upon everything with a much more discern-
ing eye. My perspective and views on so many things had changed
and what I deemed important before was now but vapor on the
wind. Now what was important were those things that could not
be touched or held on to, what was important had to be earned and
nurtured from within. My gift of Faith was a treasure more valuable
than any riches hoarded by man.

That evening I went to my prayer tree, my heart once again sagging in my chest. The footing I had on sanity earlier in the day as I sat with Faith seemed to have slipped away a bit, sending me on an emotional roller coaster ride that I wanted out of. My heart burning with pain, I asked out loud, "Do you love me? Are you there? Are you listening?" I felt those hot lava tears burn my cheeks as my heart poured forth from my eyes. I wanted to be shown that I was loved and that I could reach out and find Him when I needed to, like a child does to a parent. Without a parent to lean on, the feeling of loneliness is as vast as an ocean inside your heart. I begged for Faith's cross to be given to me to carry through life, that I would bear the weight of it for her if I could, taking on anything and everything she had to face so that she did not have to suffer. Joey came out and joined me, and together we stood under the umbrella of leaves arm in arm. We were two little people under a big tree facing big issues all alone. We only had each other for support in the vast and wild natural world. Eventually, we turned away and went to bed.

Ever felt an angel's breath in the gentle breeze? A teardrop in the falling rain? Hear a whisper amongst the rustle of leaves? Or been kissed by a lone snowflake? Nature is an angel's favorite hiding place.

~Carrie Latet~

18

In the Garden Beautiful

Gardens hold special meanings as they are a place where life is cultivated, nurtured, and tended to. There is no place quite as complete as a garden when one thinks about the cycle of organic life itself, for it is there that new life is born, growth occurs, and then death takes over for something else to be born. The four seasons can be compared to the cycle of life in a garden, spring compared to the tender young shoots we all race to plant when the signs of spring are surely in the air. Summer arrives in all her glory, and our gardens are in full swing, the bounty of their youthfulness in full blossom as they hang their ripe and sweet wares from the vine beckoning us to imbibe in the sweet juices of fruit they are offering. As fall arrives, the harvest is either complete, or the last of the fall gourds have been plucked, nature now begins her rest, peacefully wearing the crown of the fruit of her labors. When winter arrives, we mourn the loss of our bountiful gardens, for they have now passed beyond, frozen in their caskets of earth, leaving us to yearn for what was once the newness of spring that brought so much youthfulness to our hearts.

Why is it so dark in here? And then there I was, back in that heavenly room with a view. Although I couldn't see anything, I could feel the coolness of the black shelf where I could rest my arms, and again, I stood staring at nothing, waiting for the picture show to begin. I had been in this room before watching another dream-show, and now I was back to see something else materialize before my eyes. In front of me, the wall came to life, the light from the picture show glowed brightly, and inside the three-dimensional viewer, I saw the most spectacular being that I had ever seen.

My heart skipped a beat as I watched him move in and around the exotic vines and flowering bushes that grew in the garden he played in. There were utopian trees I could not identify as anything remotely similar to what was here on Earth. This being I watched moved within space and time differently than we do here in earthly time, and he played effortlessly amongst the trees as if it was pure pleasure to exist as one with nature. As I watched, spellbound, I noticed that he wasn't wearing any clothing, but no matter which way he moved, no genitals were apparent. There was nothing sexual about the nudity, and no shame existed because of the nakedness. He simply moved freely about and played in the trees, turning somersaults and laughing and smiling. He was, or seemed, totally oblivious to me as he climbed a tree. Facing sideways, he stopped with his left foot on a limb and right knee lifted up, his right foot resting on an even higher branch. It was then he seemed to notice I was watching him, and he turned and looked directly at me. Then, just as in the first dream, everything was slowed down and magnified so that every detail could be examined. The first thing I saw was his skin. It was bronze, a beautiful color that seemed as if it were lit up from within his being, and the skin itself looked as if it had been sprinkled with gold dust. His smile was brilliant white and each tooth perfectly sized and positioned within his mouth as he smiled at me. His eyes were black and his gaze so piercing that it was obvious his stare could see deep into the windows of my soul. He knew everything about me, his eyes told me that, and he still loved me anyway. He had soft, dark curls that framed his face, and his muscular physique signified strength and protection.

He loved me; I saw it in his eyes, and I felt as if he had loved me for a very long time. The feeling of love he showed me through his eyes came from within, and it wasn't a physical love he impressed upon me but a spiritual one. I blinked my eyes in disbelief at what I was seeing, and when they opened, he had come down from the tree and was standing at a distance from me with eyes still focused upon me. His smile was wide, and I blinked again; he was *this much* closer and moving closer to me! What did he want? I blinked again, and we were then face to face, staring directly into each other's eyes, separated only by the force field of the viewing screen that was between us. He intently gazed into my eyes and smiled a wide grin. I smiled back finding it a blessing to be privy to such things and stood riveted in my spot in the heavenly theater. *Do I dare even take a breath?* I thought and then blinked. With that, the scene I was viewing went dark, and he was gone; the cinema curtains had closed, and I felt the beautiful dream was over, and I felt a great disappointment come over me. FADE TO BLACK, and I slept soundly the rest of the night.

When I awoke the next morning, I felt peaceful and safe knowing once again a little piece of heaven had been revealed to me through a dream. What more could I have asked for in light of what I had asked for the night before in prayer? He did listen and answered prayers. I felt calm. Then the phone rang.

It was the hospital calling; we received the best news we could have wished for; they were ready to discharge Faith from the hospital. Faith was coming home today! Suddenly fears of new and unknown origins came calling at the doorway of my mind when I heard that news as I had just managed to get my emotions under control and now new fears appeared on the horizon for me to attempt to deal with. Now that she was coming home, would I be able to take care of her? Would I be able to administer the medications that would keep her well and out of the hospital? Tonight would be her first night at home with us, and I knew that I would stay up all night staring at her to ensure she was breathing.

When we arrived at the hospital, Faith was ready and waiting to be discharged, but before we took her home for the very first time, the hospital had to go over all her medication needs, everything we needed to do in case of an emergency and how we should protect her from germs and viruses that could inadvertently be brought into the house. For those instructions, we needed to wait for the physician on duty to come down and talk to us, and so, once again anxious feelings swirled around us. We told our nurses that Faith had never had her newborn pictures taken, something that marks a wonderful milestone in the lives of a family. The nurses promptly called the photographer for us who happened to be in the hospital that day and told us he would be up in a few moments. In the meantime, some of our nurses disappeared only to return a few minutes later to present us with a gift from all of them to Faith, and us. It was a tiny purple dress with lace and flowers on the collar complete with matching underpants. Both Joey and I broke down crying from the generosity and love they had shown us in such a time of need. That little outfit is the one she got her newborn photos taken in.

After getting all the information and documents in order, we left the hospital with a great send off, unsure of ourselves yet smiling through tears of relief that this part of the voyage was over. Now we were beginning a new leg of the journey, and having been in good hands thus far, I felt like the child whose bike had been let go of, the nurses allowing us to peddle frantically as we swerved drunkenly down the sidewalk of life. Yale had let us go but still held us close with the network of physicians they had set up for us. Waving goodbye to all of the staff who had cared for us so diligently was a bittersweet goodbye to the safety net that had protected us from those frightening feelings they had kept at bay. Now they would be gone, and it would be Joey and I who would become the only net between the top of the skyscraper and the hard asphalt road below it.

Once home, the very first thing I did was type two signs for our doors that would keep people who might suspect they were sick out of our house and away from Faith. Taping the last sign to the door, I stepped back and observed my handiwork, thinking to myself, *Mission partially complete.* With that done, we grabbed both our girls and went down to the street below and began taking pictures of each other on Faith's homecoming day in front of her sign announcing her arrival.

To me the ideal doctor would be a man endowed with profound knowledge of life and of the soul, divining any suffering or disorder of whatever kind, and restoring peace by his main presence.

~ HenriAmiel~

19

Finding and Meeting Dr. Right

The days, weeks, and months passed us by along with doctors' visits, blood work, and all that is to be expected of life in general in a house with two small children. Faith's doctor appointments were frequent and went well, and there were small adjustments made to her medication here or there. Other than that, life was smoothly moving along.

Biagio had almost completely disappeared as I only saw Faith now when I looked into her eyes. When I would change her diaper, Biagio would briefly come to mind, but then he was gone again—only coming to his mother's thoughts for a flash. Although he was disappearing, his memory would always occupy a tiny portion of my heart.

Over those seemingly normal months, I did an enormous amount of research on genital reconstructive surgery and weighed the controversial topic's pros and cons in my mind.

Pouring over anything and everything I could find on the internet, I read and re-read every piece of literature I could get my hands on. There were those who said that surgery was barbaric and called it mutilation, while others championed it saying it was the best decision to make for their child. There were two camps, those who were for and those who were against genital reconstruction. I waded through the many controversies and arguments, each side with compelling and convincing information that I had to measure to ensure whatever decision I made would be the right one for her.

Decades earlier, genital surgery was not as advanced as it had become. It left girls with no clitoris and poorly constructed external genitalia. There are many who are angry that the decision to perform surgery was done by the parents and not left up to the child to decide later on in life, as some of these women had procedures that left them both physically and mentally scarred. Then there was the camp who swore by the surgical procedure: one, if it was necessary; two, if it was done by an extremely qualified surgeon; and three, if it was done at a very early age. All of that information was a lot to digest and sort through; it created a great pressure to ensure the right decision was made.

I began by compiling two separate folders, one labeled *pro* and one labeled *con*, and began to search for a way to get in touch with other parents. I found a website that also functioned as a forum for parents and those who were affected by this disorder. It was a place to go and voice your opinions and thoughts, and to find support from other people who had the experience to guide you through any questions you may have. Then there was the CARES Foundation which stands for **C**ongenital **A**drenal hyperplasia, **R**esearch, **E**ducation, and **S**upport which I found to be a great source of information for me, and so, after reading what was on the site, I contacted the founder. She was a wonderful woman who managed the foundation so she could assist those who suffer with this condition. She was very quick to get back in touch with me and guided me through a lot of my concerns. She put me in touch with parents who had opted to have surgery done, and those who had opted to wait until later so that Joey and I could hear both opinions from families like ours. In the meantime, we talked, read, did research, and posted questions on the message board online. We thought about the decision for weeks on our own and together, to hear each other's personal thoughts and concerns on the topic. We felt it was wise to think of this decision both alone and together, with the support of the CARES Foundation as the first few days after finding everything out was sheer chaos within the town. By separating our thoughts from one another, a more clear and concise view of our own opinions could be formed. We did not want to sway each other should our opinions and concerns be different. Instead, we wanted to ensure we heard each other out and weighed each other's opinions with an open mind. After studying and managing everything that had been placed in front of us, we realized we were both in the same camp. Faith was so severely virilized that surgical reconstruction would be necessary as soon as possible. It was then again we turned to the CARES Foundation for gentle words, support and willingness to hold us in their arms as we movied forward with our decision.

My fears and concerns weren't at the forefront of the decision; it was her well-being, medical needs, and what she would have to endure later that made my decision a clear one. She would need surgery at some point before she began menstruating. For this, we felt that anything that needed to be done should be done early enough to minimize the psychological effects she may experience if it were put off until later in life. Next, finding a qualified surgeon to perform this delicate surgery was the hurdle to overcome. The feeling being that with the surgery so intricate to be performed, someone who had done one or two in their career was not going to be qualified to operate on our child needing such extensive work. So, we pressed the help of our pediatrician to find us Dr. Right.

Americans search long and hard for our vehicles and electronics, yet for the most part, we put our trust in those who have fancy letters that read MD behind their names. There is something about that kind of knowledge that seems to lull us into complacency. However, for my daughter, I figured that there must be every range of quality out there in doctors from fantastically qualified to not so great. For her I wanted fantastic, especially when it came to having to deal with the delicate nature of the subject matter, and I wanted the best one to be had.

Once again, Dr. Williams pulled through for us finding the name of a highly qualified surgeon very close to us in New York City. As well, the CARES Foundation also mentioned this surgeon, pushing some worries away. I couldn't believe the odds of that happening; I was expecting Timbuktu located in the East Outer Limits as my choice of surgeons, but I got New York instead, which was great news because it wasn't very far away from us. *Thank you, God!* I prayed. *There are miracles everywhere.* After scheduling appointments, we waited for the day to go to New York for our first one.

Joey had family members who had offered to help our family out in the household chores. Joey's father and wife also accompanied us to the train station to support us any way they could. The appointment scheduled to see the urologist was a few days away. They waited for my sister to arrive, then left shortly after. She had flown into New York then caught the train into New Haven. Ruth, Faith, Joe, and I had driven to the train station to greet her, and we hugged and kissed each other through tears. It had been a couple of years since I had last seen my sister, so this moment in time was a moment marked, with her holding Ruth and remarking how big she had gotten. She then took a quiet moment to peek in on Faith who was slumbering in her stroller. My sister's tears fell as she kissed Faith's swollen cheeks, the sheer gravity of it hitting her now that Faith was more than a baby babbling on the telephone. We must have stayed at the train station for over an hour just sitting and talking before realizing that time had slipped by, so we all headed home for some much-needed rest.

I was feeling the stress of things again as I needed to have all my ducks in a row as far as questions or concerns to ensure I had my questions answered while I was there on my consultation with Dr. Right. I had been writing questions down as they came to me for several weeks and had everything I wanted to bring with me in a satchel. In order to see this doctor, I would also have to see the endocrinologist that was considered to be the world's leading expert on CAH.

I had gone to doctors all my life and never felt intimidated or overwhelmed by the thought of having to speak to them, but knowing that I would have to see doctors with such big and fancy titles was frightening, to say the least. Also, these doctors were, in essence, the end of the line; the buck stopped here with them. They didn't come any better than this. There were no better doctors to see after them, and their opinions were the best opinions we were going to get. Ever. Anywhere. In the whole wide world.

And then the time was upon us. Three days later we arrived at the hospital where she would have surgery. We wound our way through the maze of elevators and floors until we came to the doctor's office. We sat outside the doors in the hallway, and it was still early in the morning, and so, the office wasn't open yet. Soon, more and more people with small children, medium-sized children, and big children began arriving, all lining up late like mourning doves on a wire. We were a pathetic pack of parents sitting there on our benches with children of all ages and sizes waiting to see the guru of glands. My nerves began to get the better of me, and once again, to escape the anxiety of waiting to meet this doctor, my imagination entertained me. In my mind's eye I could see her riding in on her pachyderm or escorted by men in turbans who were wearing beautifully designed regalia. She didn't talk or walk. Or maybe her residents carried her in a palanquin adorned and bejeweled with riches beyond imagination. I mean, she was a prominent, fancy doctor, and this was a well-known hospital, after all. But when the doors opened and my appointment came, I saw a person much different than the one I envisioned. The doctor was a mature woman who was extremely knowledgeable and professional, not the exotic image of a bejeweled doctor, wearing exotic scarves, and a medicine woman, who specialized in unusual ailments that I conjured up.

In the usual, very special fashion of being a very special doctor, she had her very special residents swarming around her in her very special office, listening to her very special words and doing everything that the very special doctor asked. It was hot in the examination room with the doctor. The residents, my sister, Joey, Ruth, and I were clinging to the side of the wall like spiders ogling Faith, who had inadvertently landed in a web. I wanted out of there as fast as my legs could carry me, but we still had other items on the agenda before we could go home. The examination included the usual diaper check where the diaper would quickly come off so everyone could get a gander at the little girl's pee-pee parts, which I quickly put a stop to all together. Blood work needed to be taken and determined by the magic eight ball where the fortune of lab work arrives with answers for the exceptional doctor's professional advice. Her advice was comprised of a plethora of valuable information. She then advised me to take her recommendations back to the physicians that cared for Faith in Connecticut. After about thirty minutes, the examination was over. I stepped into the hallway with a sigh of relief and then moved to the next leg of the expedition.

The urologist was next on our agenda, and once in his office, I looked around at all the other parents in the room. What were the ailments their infants were struggling with? Why were they here? Was it something simple for them, or was it something more complex than even we were facing? There were people from all walks of life waiting to see this man, some appeared quite wealthy and some did not. *An individual so wise and well known as this doctor must be about a hundred years old and hunched over from years of performing the same surgery night and day*, I thought to myself. I imagined him to be wearing thick bifocal glasses from the strain of millions of precision cuts and stitches, worn to the scalp was his hair in a Nutty Professor style. Anyone this smart and this busy would surely have no cares about appearance or have any time to maintain them. I could see this old curmudgeon moving from examining room to examining room by means of shuffling his feet, one foot in an orthopedic shoe with a five-inch lift on it which slowed him down by banging down noisily every time he shuffle-stepped in front of the other foot. Laughing to myself, I took a quick look around the office again, seeing many nurses coming and going into the bustling office each with their own task to do. There was a man standing at the desk talking into a recorder and a receptionist assisting patients with their appointments. Everyone performed their job in this very special office for this very special doctor who specialized in very special surgeries.

Bernadette and I exchanged small talk while keeping an eye on Faith and watching Ruth play in the waiting room as we waited. Joey sat quietly, taking in everything, and sensing his worry and anticipation, I put my arm around him in support as he had always been there for me. I told him that everything would be fine. He nodded yes, smiled, and then looked away again, distant and deep in thought. "I can't wait to see this guy," I said exuberantly to him, hoping to engage him in conversation to get his mind away from itself. "Me too, Kaye. I'm really anxious to see what he has to say," he answered back quietly.

Our day had already been peppered with long waits and blood drawn at the other doctor's office, and I hoped that it wouldn't be the same experience here. But soon after our arrival, our appointment time rolled around, and they called us into an examining room where my sister took her spot on a windowsill next to the exam table. Joey and I took the two chairs in the room, and Ruth rested in Joey's lap while I held Faith. Five minutes later, the door opened, and the doctor appeared in the room. Surprisingly, it was the same man I saw talking into the recorder at the desk in the waiting room. He was not old at all, and quite frankly, I was disappointed to see that he was as young as he was. How could he be qualified when he was too young to have that kind of experience under his belt? But there he stood and introduced himself as the very special doctor we had come all the way from Connecticut to see.

I identified myself as Faith's mother and placed her on the exam table. He asked us to remove her diaper so that he could examine her, and after he did, he took a seat and began to speak.

He went over every aspect of the surgery and the debate over reconstructive surgery that we needed to know about. He left no detail out, taking his time to ensure that we understood exactly what he was telling us. He covered both sides of the surgical debate, laying everything on the table for us to hear. The information he shared was spooned to us in terms we could understand, and the whole time he spoke he sat next to the exam table with his hand on Faith's tummy. I squirmed in my seat at the uncomfortable nature of the conversation; however, the conversation was necessary. Furthermore, it needed to be spoken so we as parents had all the information lined up in front of us. This very special doctor wasn't going to do any very special surgery, on any very special child or person, without all the very special facts put on the table.

I broke down and cried at the information as I found some of it confusing to wade through, yet he never stopped giving the facts to us, one after the other, laying it out in black and white, never flinching at our reactions. We asked our questions, me, Joey, and Bernadette, to which he answered every one of them honestly. The subject of surgery on Faith came up, and he informed us that he preferred to do this type of surgery early, and if we opted for surgery, he would prefer to do Faith's at around four months of age. We agreed and chose to have everything done at once so it would be the last time she went in for a major surgery of this type and it would be over and done with. He stood and shook Joey's hand, said his goodbyes to my sister and I and then turned around, one hand on his chin, looking at Faith. He stood there for some time, then shook his head ever so slightly and walked out of the door.

We scheduled another appointment with him as he needed to do some preliminary procedures on Faith before surgery to get an understanding of how everything appeared inside of her. From what I could gather, it was a way of mapping out the route he would take during surgery, so he would already have a plan when he went in to do battle. He would eventually become my General MacArthur, mapping out strategies of how to master the battlefield and conquer each unfamiliar territory explored. But now, I was overwhelmed and tired. We left in silence, each of us holding on to our own thoughts and impressions as we made our way back to the main level of the hospital. My mind was racing, *Boys, girls, girls, boys, male parts that aren't, female parts that are, virilized, do the surgery, don't do the surgery, wait, proceed, fertility, medicine, blood work, bone age, lifetime, blah, blah, blah!* And then I heard, "He's the man you want," my sister said coming up behind me and then walked away, leaving me with that one thought.

Riding home, I thought about our visit and him, the urologist who gave me everything he had during the appointment. He unloaded, leaving no stone unturned, and all that information burned hotly in my ears and pierced my mind with the evidence I needed to make a well-informed decision. I liked that, but even more, I liked the fact that he never took his hand off of my daughter. His focus, although informing us of everything we needed to know, was on Faith. There was no one in the room that was more important than her, and it was his actions coupled with his words that validated that for me. Very special doctor had become Dr. Right and restored peace to my soul about the decision. I turned to my sister and said, "You know what, he *is* the man I want, the ideal doctor," and with that, we all agreed and talked about him, Faith, and our visit the rest of the way home.

Prayers go up, and blessings come down.

~Yiddish Proverb~

20

A Baptism Amid Chaos

Bernadette's visit had come and gone, and the fall season was quickly moving in on us. Faith's surgery was right around the corner, and we needed to have her baptized before the surgery date. Ramona would be her godmother, and Joey's childhood friend Bobby would be her godfather. Mona was in Virginia on business and would be catching a flight up to be in attendance at the baptism. I had gotten up early that morning and dropped Ruth off at our neighborhood daycare, as I had a lot of last-minute arrangements to accomplish. First, though, I would need my morning dose of news and a cup of coffee.

There are those particular events in your life that are so shocking, the news of them can shake you to the core of your being. There are also those life-changing events that are so disturbing they disrupt the very air you breathe. Take for instance, the untimely death of Princess Diana, who died in a horrific crash in a tunnel in Paris. I remember exactly where I was when I heard the news. I was working, unlocking the door as employees entered for their daily shift.

In 2001, we began planning out Faith's baptism, and the date would be coming soon. I awoke one morning to watch my favorite news channel and was taken aback by what I was seeing. Planes flying into the World Trade Center buildings and chaos happening everywhere. Then it happened, the Pentagon and Somerset County in Pennsylvania. I held my breath, so frightened. I put Faith in her bassinet and went to the front door to look out into the sky. *Are they coming here? Was this a massive attack on all of America?* I stared for quite some time until Joey called me to see if we were okay. He was on his way to pick up a generator and grab Ruth from daycare to bring home so we could all be together. That brought comfort amidst the chaos that was taking place in "real" time.

I so selfishly said a small prayer, I thought, *Lord, please don't let our surgeon be in one of those buildings. Faith's surgery is only four days away. What will I do without him, and what will the world do without all the special people who are lost?* This was a heartbreaking moment in time to live through, and this heartbreaking moment in time still lives on. I would need to call my sister to see if she knew how we were going to handle the baptism.

I called Ramona to let her know what was happening. I pulled her out of her meeting to inform her that there were no flights and she probably wouldn't make it up to attend the baptism. However, knowing my sister's tenacity, I had a feeling she would find a way, and sure enough, she did. She found one of the last rental cars available and drove herself up to be with us. It was one of the sweetest, let alone luckiest, thing my sister had done for me.

The day of the baptism had arrived amidst the chaos going on in the world, and although still nervous, we continued. Once the ceremony was over, we went to the hall rented for celebration, but there, in the air, still hung the cloak of sadness that had enveloped all of America.

"If you look deeply into the palm of your hand, you will see your parents and all generations of your ancestors. All of them are alive in this moment. Each is present in your body. You are the continuation of each of these people."

~Thich Nhat Han~

21

The Gatekeepers

I was a really young girl when my mother died. So young that I had not developed the maturity to have had those adult conversations adult children must undoubtedly have with their parents at some particular point in their lives. There were no questions pointed to my mother as to why's, or where's, or who's, or what's for me. My focus was on the future, as to how I was going to survive the aftermath of her death, and coping in the present with the daily routine of attending to her needs. I was also more concerned with being a teenager at that time in my life and the blossoming young person I was becoming than what my past could teach me about my history, my ancestors, and myself.

When my mother died, a vacuum of empty space filled the depression where she once lived and breathed. There was no grandmother, grandfather, mother, or father to fill the void. No one to assist or guide me into womanhood, no one to tell me where I was going, and no one to tell me where I came from. When my mother escaped the confines of this physical world, so, too, did the *her*story of me that was carried away with her.

When a mother dies prematurely, a vast library of information goes with her, and if there are no historians left to enlighten the young one once they are big enough to listen with a purpose. That young person becomes adrift on a vast ocean, caught in the doldrums on a dinghy, drifting from current to current, searching for their multifaceted identity.

It took me a long time to mature into an adult because of the lack of a mother, but what I learned through this life lesson was that I had sisters, other extensions of family that could function as historians to me. Maybe not like mother could, but for some of those unanswered questions that hovered aimlessly in my mind, my sisters were able to fill in the blanks, one conversation at a time. I didn't even think to ask them until I had gotten older, and now that this situation had arisen, little tidbits of information surfaced that I would have never known about. Like the church for one, and many other little stories and anecdotes my sisters had shared with me through lengthy conversations. Because there was such a huge difference in age between myself and the rest of my siblings, in many aspects, being the youngest was like being an only child. I didn't have the same sibling relationship as someone shares with a sibling close to them in age. My sisters were the gatekeepers for a life and time I otherwise would not have had any answers to.

The lesson here is that no matter how far life may take you from those you love, the bonds of family are much deeper than just the love itself that ties you all together. It is the "who" that carries the depth of importance. If you know nothing about yourself, where you came from, who your ancestors were, and what your cultural background is, then you know nothing about the face that peers back at you in the mirror. When you look at your image in the mirror, it should come alive; through your eyes, you should see all of those who made you ripple and move beneath your skin. You are the manifestation of all of those relatives and ancestors who came before you, and all of them have a story to tell that is part of the fabric of your DNA. All of them can whisper your history to you collectively if you listen hard enough, weaving the historical bonds of family so tightly together that no matter the reason for separation, be it time or distance, exactly *who* you are will never be in question.

As a result, I have now become the active gatekeeper, the literary shaman of family stories, such as medical information, anecdotes, births, deaths, tragedies and triumphs to tell my daughters. I write down as much information as I can recall. I rely on my own gatekeepers to open the floodgates and let their remembrances flow freely to me, and from me to the pen, and from the pen to the paper. Now their *her*story will be preserved and written down, kept safe for them so that when my daughters do peer into their own hands, the pages of my journals shall come alive with the voices of their ancestors, and nothing of the knowledge of those ancestors I have gained will have been lost when I pass away.

Every man is a quotation from all his ancestors

~Ralph Waldo Emmerson~

Dare to reach out your hand into the darkness, to pull another hand into the light.

~Norman B. Rice~

22

A Surgeon's Hands

Have you ever felt like time stood still? I have, on several monumental occasions in my life, and today was another one of those moments where time would tick by, then stop, leaving me feeling the movement of my body still in motion while the world itself had jerked to a standstill. Today was the eve of Faith's surgery, and we were sailing out on yet another voyage that would put us in uncharted territory as parents. I thought about all the moments leading up to this point and how we, as a family, had been taken to the mountaintop, to the crest of a wave and peered down the other side where easy traversing and smooth sailing awaited us. We weren't there yet, but soon we would be, and with every step we took, it brought us closer to the finish line. I would be fine one minute, and the next, I would be lost in a sea of dark emotions pitting decisions and fear of the unknown against each other. Time ticked by, sometimes gracing me with calming thoughts that made everything okay in the world. The next minute, electricity would be coursing through my veins as everything stopped except for me, leaving me emotionally catapulting forward out of a trebuchet with nothing dead ahead but a brick wall to stop me. I had second-guessed myself on numerous occasions, and as the surgical date grew near, my nerves became raw and chafed, causing me to bristle at everything.

I would check all of my facts over and over again, scrutinizing details inch by inch, ensuring everything was in order, not wanting any oversights or missteps to occur. I crossed every "T" and dotted every "I" until I was sure that I was comfortable with the fact that this was the right decision. Today, time was playing games with me, letting me know that no matter what I did or how I felt, nothing could change the fact that it would continue to tick, tock on, in a countdown to send my child off in the care of a stranger's hands. Those thoughts of what she might think when she got older dangled in my mind, guilt parading back and forth, salivating from his handy work. The overall decision was a very hard one as there was so much controversy to be had on both sides of the issue. I did what I felt was ultimately the right thing for her, not me, and so I knew that I must push past all the maternal worries I was bombarding myself with. All I focused on was the thought that we must move forward with the decision made knowing that it wouldn't have been made had it not been the right one in the first place.

Mona had already returned to California, and this morning I particularly wished for my sisters, both or either one, to have been able to be here with me through the procedure. As well, going into New York after 9/11 was nerve-wracking; we weren't sure what we would see or even knew how safe it was going to be there. I packed Faith's favorite blue blanket that Ruth had given to her. It was the one she slept with every night. I had also made a little mobile with all of our pictures on it so that Faith would always see pictures of her family around her no matter who was in the room with her. I took with me a packet of stationary and a Bible, assuming any other reading material I might want could be found in the gift shop. Then we were ready, kind of, sort of, almost. There was one more thing I needed to do, and that was to take a picture of Faith on the eve of her surgery. I wanted this day of transition recorded for her, a day that signified a change that would metamorphosize the current tide into an ocean of difference. I propped her up in bed with Ruth, and danced around until they laughed, and I snapped the photo of them laughing, her, oblivious to the events that were unfolding in front of her. This was a poignant time for me as I loved her no matter what, no matter how she was packaged, and I promised her that no secrets would be kept from her, that she would know all there was to know about her condition when she was old enough to understand. I would owe her that respect; she deserved that from me and deserved to know the details of our struggle with making some of the hardest decisions of our lives for her. This was a moment when time stood still for me again. A strange, wistful feeling evaded my soul, and tears welled up in my eyes. Today would be the very last day I would see her the way she had been sent to me from above, as I had grown accustomed to seeing her just as she was gifted to our family. Tomorrow would bring yet another change, for her, the incredible changing baby that continued to emerge as a new butterfly from its chrysalis, growing more precious and more beautiful each and every day.

Arriving in New York just a few hours after we left our home, we checked into the hotel next door to the hospital. It was a hotel that had been recommended to us since the Ronald McDonald House was full. It was a place where many families stayed while waiting for a loved one to have and recover from surgery, and we found it quite comfortable and convenient for our needs. We settled in and quickly went over the plans we had discussed before we made the trip over to the hospital to check Faith in. The hotel was literally right next door, so the walk over wouldn't take long at all; however, when we started to make the short trip to the hospital for check-in, my feet became heavy, and I grew anxious. Knowing that Faith would be separated from us again was a tough thought to process as it *felt* like she had only been home with us for a few short weeks.

The check-in went smoothly, and Faith was placed in her room where we were given specific instructions not to feed her after seven that evening. Although I knew that we weren't going to be able to feed her, hearing it made me panic, so Joey agreed to take this first shift, knowing I would have a very hard time not feeding her. I accepted, and took Ruth back to the hotel with me to get sleep if I could before the morning marathon began. My night's sleep was fitful, and the next morning came before I knew it, but I was up in a flash getting the both of us ready well before the sun came up.

At the hospital an hour later, I found Joey going over the schedule with his father and his father's wife who had come to offer their support to us by helping with Ruth as we waited for Faith's surgery to be completed. Joey greeted both Ruth and I with hugs and kisses and told me that the night had gone well and that Faith had slept soundly. I was relieved to hear that news, and we sat for a few minutes talking amongst the four of us with Ruth on my lap and Faith in my arms. Then, before I knew it, there was a tap at the door, and I saw that the team had arrived and were coming to prepare my Faith for surgery. They entered the room, moving about, looking at charts, wristbands, etcetera in preparation for what was to come, and another nurse scanned the room looking for me, the mother, and said in a very comforting tone, "It's time." I took a deep breath and nodded my head slowly up and down, acknowledging that I was on board and ready as well. One nurse asked who would be carrying Faith into the operating room, and

Joey pointed to me, knowing I wouldn't have it any other way. I needed to have my hands on her until I wasn't able to anymore. Then they handed me a white jumpsuit that resembled a nuclear hazmat suit, which I would have to wear to take Faith into the operating room. I put the suit on and began to feel the incredible crush of weight that was pressing down on me. With tears welling up in my eyes, I picked up my sweet Faith and began what felt like was going to be a long walk down a long corridor to the electric chair. Joey and I said our goodbyes to everyone in the room and allowed Ruth to kiss her sister goodbye. Then the three of us moved out of the door and into the hallway with the one remaining nurse who had stayed with us.

The walk was a long and winding one, taking us to the farthest outposts of the hospital where not many people go, stopping when we reached a bank of elevators that would take us to our destination. At the elevator, the nurse told Joey he could not go any further with Faith, and would have to say goodbye here. Now, mother and daughter were to go the rest of the way together. Joey kissed her goodbye and stood there to wait for me to return as the door on the elevator closed. His face was a stark reminder to me of what still lay before us. I went on holding Faith as tight as I could, escorted by the nurse who was leading the way down, down, down to the operating room.

Once in the elevator, the woman began to engage me in small talk about the surgery. During the conversation, she asked me how I found out about this doctor, and I told her. She then told me that if it were her daughter that needed this type of surgery, he would be the surgeon she would choose. She went on to tell me that Faith was in the best of hands and would be taken good care of. I assumed the kind words were to put me at ease, and I certainly appreciated their calming effects. However, I already knew he was the best there was to be found. Anywhere. In the whole wide, wide world.

The woman escorted me to the door of the operating room, and when the door opened, I was greeted by a blast of hot air. I peered in tentatively and noticed the room had a blue monochrome color scheme to it. I observed a long table at one end of the room that had been draped with a cloth, and lined up neatly on top of it were surgical instruments that I assumed were going to be used in the surgery. Those did not look like ordinary surgical instruments (not that I knew what ordinary surgical instruments looked like), but these things looked like they cost something special.

You know how it is. Like when we were young and would go over to a friend's house to eat supper because they were having steak. Mrs. So-n-so would pan fry the cheapest cut of steak there was and serve it up with a butter knife. Then you would spend the rest of dinner chasing that overcooked piece of shoe leather around the plate with a knife and fork, drooling and working hard for each morsel of steak you struggled to saw through with those worn out knives. Then there was the chef who had his own, specialized, personalized cooking tools. This doctor's tools were not in the category of everyday household utensil category, they were in the "I'm a chef, and I only use the finest shit" category.

In the operating room there were a number of people, all of whom were wearing blue scrubs and masks buzzing about, doing different tasks while the woman I was with instructed me to walk inside the room and lay Faith down on the table. Faith, clad only in a diaper, was looking around the room taking everything in without a care in the world, oblivious to what was going to take place. A masked person standing at the head of the table put a clear mask on her face, and I watched my little girl twitch once as her eyes rolled back in her head, and her entire body relaxed. Her arms fell limply down to her sides, and her little head rolled over to one side. The last thing I saw was her two little white teeth sticking out of her open mouth before I was tapped on the shoulder. I looked up, and another masked person told me that she was asleep and that it was time to leave. I stared at the face for a moment before realizing that it was the surgeon himself signaling for me to go. I could tell by his eyes that he was smiling at me as he told me she was in good hands and not to worry. I nodded yes and turned to walk out before I started crying. I was scared, and I wanted my mother, or sisters, or one of them, if not all, to be with me right then and there. It was over now, and all I could do was wait until the surgery was over to see her again.

As frightening as it was to watch the process of Faith being put to sleep, I was fascinated by it at the same time. The little mask that was placed over her face seemed to hover there for a second or two, and then it was all over. She was out like a light after breathing in the magic gas from the magic dragon's hookah. One breath and she was awake; the next, she was in some other world. Anytime we are ever in the operating room it is usually because we are the ones on the table. To actually *see* the process of being administered anesthesia is fascinating. I could not get over how fast she went from reacting to being put on the table, her little arms and legs wiggling around, to seconds later being limp and lifeless. Today I had the unique perspective of being that gnat on the southside wall watching all the very special worker bees prepare for a surgery in a room that seemed to have electricity pulsing through the air as everyone focused on what they needed to accomplish.

From the operating room, I met back up with Joey again, and we were escorted to what seemed to be an out of the way waiting room where we would be able to get updates on how the surgery was progressing by a nurse in the operating room. The in-laws took

Ruth and headed back to the hotel room while Joey and I stayed and waited and waited and waited. This waiting served a purpose for me, reflection. I sat and reflected on all the things that had taken place to lead up to this moment, and my decision was taking place in a room somewhere in the hospital. My thoughts were also on the man whom I had put all of my trust into, and as my thoughts fell on him and the task he was faced with, I knew I needed to pray. I found my way down to the chapel where I prayed for a long while. My prayers were not for the surgery to be over quickly and all those other purposeful things we pray about in our scripted prayers, but one that put him at the center of my intentions. My prayers were for the surgeon, asking that *he* be blessed in his work and that his hands be guided in the most skillful manner to do the work he was put here on Earth to do. My other prayer would be for him and his team that they be blessed. I had reached out into the unknown darkness, reaching for the surgeon's hands and pulling them into the light.

The rest of the wait was an arduous one with the hours ticking by and Joey and I growing increasingly restless. It seemed like forever, sitting there in the non-specific room with non-specific paint on the walls and non-specific chairs that turned on you after sitting in them for more than thirty minutes at a clip, biting at your hips and gnawing on your backbone. Time and all its trickery seemed to have stood still again but only within the confines of this stale room, leaving us to steep in stagnant thoughts while the rest of the world continued on, oblivious to what was unfolding inside the building.

Eventually the surgery came to an end, and we were instructed to go to a set of elevators and wait for the doctor who would come out and give us the details of the surgery. It was over, and Faith was being moved into the recovery room where we could see her. Excited, Joey rushed over to the elevator and waited for the doctor, and I went to find my father-in-law, his wife, and Ruth. Returning empty handed, he told me I had missed the doctor who said that everything went very well and that Faith did not need all of the surgical procedures he thought she was going to, likening her surgery to a haircut. He told Joey it was more like trimming a head of hair than restyling one. I immediately broke down into tears, so happy at the news that my little one, once again, had kicked ass in her very short life. She went into surgery like a little trooper and came out the other end showing the well-seasoned and very experienced surgeon things he had not seen before. *Yeah, Mom,* I thought, *you would be proud of her.* Soon thereafter, a nurse came out to get us telling us we could come into the recovery room to see her. We stood stiffly, almost afraid to move, afraid to see what we might see yet excited to see our sweet baby girl again.

Once inside the recovery room, the nurse pointed to the corner where she was, and I began to grow nervous because I could see her tiny body lying motionless in the corner next to the nurses' station. But as I got closer, I could see she was still asleep as the anesthesia had not completely worn off. Just seeing her lying there made me cry, and I began to feel anxiety at what I was going to see. I could picture myself with that B-rated movie's terror-stricken face as they removed her bandages. Black and white film, me with my hands on my cheeks, my face frozen in fear, screaming at what was being revealed as they pulled each bandage away. I had no idea what she was going to look like now, and I was very hesitant to see. What were we going to see? What was she going to look like? Would she function properly after this complicated surgery? I hesitantly walked behind Joey, and we were led over to where she was. The nurse closed the curtain so that we could have some privacy, and Joey and I laughingly noted that she looked like a porcelain doll in a box. She was lying perfectly still on her back with a blanket neatly tucked over her chest and under her arms. Her plump arms were placed neatly by her sides, and her little face was as still as could be. I leaned over and kissed her as the nurse folded back the blanket to show us the surgeon's work. Over the genitals was another little piece of gauze, I don't quite remember as the moment was a bit surreal. The nurse gently lifted it up, and I could hear my heart pounding rapidly in my ears as I steadied myself in preparation to view what the surgeon had done. And then it was revealed. She was simply... perfect. If I didn't know any better, I would have thought that she was born that way. I was more than amazed at the transformation that had occurred inside that superheated room by the hands of a surgeon whose dedication to patients both large and small far surpassed anything I had ever witnessed. I took a step back in disbelief and sat down, weeping once again with relief that everything was over, and judging by the information relayed to Joey, the internal work that needed to be done went more than well. Joey and I hugged each other and smiled, and then I left the recovery room so that Joey's father could come and join him at her bedside.

I have to say there is no feeling like the release of stress after getting the best news of your life, and after spending those few moments in the recovery room, I felt as if the weight of the world had been lifted from my shoulders now that this leg of the journey was behind us. After being "shooed" out of recovery, we all enjoyed a nice meal in Manhattan courtesy of Joseph Sr., and his wife and then said our goodbyes to them as they headed back to Connecticut. Joey, Ruth, and I were spent and needed a good night's rest, but first, we all needed to make some phone calls to let friends and family know that the surgery had gone well. After those phone calls, we made our way back to the hospital to check in on Faith, only to find that she had been moved to a special observation room where she would remain until morning. We stayed for a while, keeping vigil over her one at a time as we had to keep watch over Ruth as well. Eventually, we were shooed away from there, too, the nurses knowing there was nothing we could do for her there and that we had had a very long day and needed rest. We took them up on it and wearily walked back to the hotel together, a tired family who had been through all together.

The next couple of days were spent running back and forth to the hospital, watching Ruth, and having our blood work done for genetic testing. Ruth had also requested to see her sister and was told that they would accommodate her request. Once again, Ruth was *only* allowed to see her through a window. When Ruth saw her lying in her bed, she waved hello and blew her a kiss, but seeing Faith hooked up to machines with tubing running in and around her must have been too much for her. Ruth became quite talkative and seemed to grow more and more upset as we left the area where Faith was. Eventually she became so jittery that she vomited in the corridor of the hospital and began to cry for her sister to come home. I felt terrible as there is nothing that can prepare you as a mother for the circumstances of having a child in the hospital and another one who is struggling to understand what is going on around them. I was at a complete loss as to how to handle the situation but did the best I knew how. I took her back to the hotel room and comforted her by talking to her about what upset her in two-year-old talk. She told me she wanted "Cake" home and was scared to see her behind the "glass wall." I told her that "Cake" would be coming home soon and that they would be able to do a lot of things together just like all sisters do. That seemed to make her feel better, but the reference to "Cake" was a first since her prediction some time ago.

Millions of spiritual creatures walk the earth unseen,
both when we wake and when we sleep.

~ **John Milton,** *Paradise Lost* ~

23

His Angels Are in the Wind

The week in the hospital was a long and arduous one with many doctors coming in and out, poking and prodding Faith and discussing the surgery with Joey and I. Faith had been put in what they called a mermaid wrap, which was nothing more than ace bandages wrapped around both of her legs so that she would remain immobile. Try as they might, they could not keep her in that wrap for anything. She would raise her legs high in the air like they were being hoisted up on a pulley and then tip them forward over her head. Then, with all her might, she would raise herself straight up in the air, lifting her little butt off the mattress like she was going to do a reverse headstand and then slam her legs down on the mattress until she could free herself of the wrap. No matter how many times I would re-wrap the bandage, which, by the way, she would lay perfectly still and allow me to do, she would become Houdini and escape from her bindings. Then I would cringe as she would grab her toes and pull her legs apart as babies do, touching her toes to the mattress on each side of her. Sometimes she would put her toes in her mouth, both of them at the same time, and look at me with a little devilish look and smile at me as she munched happily on her toes. I wondered if that hurt, but she never displayed any signs of pain. An interesting side note: To this day, Faith loves magic, especially the escape artist Houdini. Despite the bruising and stitches, this feisty little girl just wanted free of her wrap to wriggle around in her crib. She was a fighter, and her spirit shined through during her recovery in the hospital. She laughed and played and smiled through it all, and once a full week had gone by, we were able to take her home with us.

Before we knew it, life had simply returned to normal for us. We attended church, took walks in the park together, and began the healing process, knowing that the hardest part of all of this was finally over. The six months following the surgery progressed quite well, and she was almost a year old, and as of yet, we had not been hit by any serious illness accompanied by a fever. I really enjoyed this first year with her, and albeit a tough one, she had brought me so much joy.

One of my favorite things was for her to wake me in the middle of the night by clicking her tongue. She wouldn't cry, rather she would "click, click, click," her tongue until I would wake up. It was a pleasant way to be roused out of a dead sleep instead of a jolting cry. One night she woke me up clicking, and as I picked her up, I immediately realized she was burning up. My heart nearly jumped out of my mouth as I knew I was going to have to put into action everything I had been taught by the doctors so long ago. My mind began to race, *What was I supposed to do? Take her temperature; what do I do? What if the temperature is above a certain temperature? I double the dose; if it is over that level, then I triple the dose? Oh, come on, Kaye, remember!* I got Joey up out of bed, and we began to go over all the information we needed to remember. First, take her temperature and then try to get the fever down to normal. "Oh my gosh, she just vomited!" I nervously said to Joey, and now we were both in full panic mode. Within fifteen minutes she had vomited again. I gave her a dose of her steroid to compensate for the fever and hovered over her crib, staring at her like my eyes would send out laser beams to remove the virus or bacteria that had made her sick. Fifteen minutes later she vomited again, and the fever was still going strong, not backing down to children's fever medication, cool cloths, nothing. Not wanting to take any more of a chance, we packed our bags and headed out the door with Ruth in tow to the emergency room at Yale.

Once there, they took immediate action in caring for her, and we sat helplessly by watching as they hovered over her, giving her an IV, and asking us questions about her. As I held her, they took her temperature, and it registered at 102 degrees! All sorts of worries began to circulate in my mind. *Would they be able to lower the fever?* I wondered. I was sweating with fear over what would happen to her if they could not get the fever to break. I watched helplessly as she shrieked and wailed in my arms, her little body stiff as a board and hot and sweaty with the embers that burned inside her. I wasn't sure what to expect that night and was very fearful that she was going to have an adrenal crisis and die in my arms.

I suppose it was the fear of experiencing the dreaded fever for the first time, this I can say for sure. It was one of the moments in my life when those old feelings of fear took hold of me. The pain of my mother's death loomed over me, and I became paralyzed with it at the thought of having no control over losing a second loved one to an illness once again in my life. I hated that helpless feeling because it forced me to realize just how small I really was in the bigger picture of the world.

If you have ever taken a trip to Sequoia National Park and stood at the foot of General Sherman, one of the largest trees in the world, then you know what I am referring to in the realm of control. That tree is an experience unlike any other. It is nature's cathedral, and as you stand there, the realization of just how small we are in comparison to the earth becomes crystal clear. Gazing up into the tree's canopy you are in absolute awe of its magnificence, and it lets you know there is a much greater force at work that we humans have no control over. Despite our great medical and technological advances, if it is our time to pass beyond, we do not have the choice to decide otherwise.

Choking back my fears, I sang to her, rocked her, and walked with her the best I could, waiting and praying that whatever the concoction was inside the IV it would help lower the wildfire that was raging inside her. It worked, bringing her fever down a bit, quieting her down into a fitful sleep on my shoulder. She and I would be spending the night in the hospital, and Joey and Ruth would go home together. I kissed my little sleeping Ruth goodnight, and Joey took her home, and then I went upstairs with Faith where I would sit up for the most part of the night keeping vigil beside her crib.

Eventually her fever subsided, and I was able to relax enough to get a little sleep. Before I did, I thought about this last event and felt that the last hurdle in learning about this condition had passed us through the thicket. Getting through the fever was the last thing we had to experience to complete the entire lap of all there was to complete in learning about this condition, and now we had finally done so. Thank goodness! Now we would know what to expect and how to handle it without being half as frightened the next time around.

The following morning, Faith was fine, and with that came her discharge from the hospital. Faith's fever had broken the night before, and she was back to her old self again, waking me with her click, click, clicking of the tongue. Her oversized cheeks were rosy, and her eyes were alert and full of life. I felt so happy to see her wiggling around in the crib like nothing had ever happened. Exhausted from the night before, I felt a great sense of peace wash over me as I reflected on the year I had experienced since her birth.

It was a powerful thought to think that my personal growth had come so far in so many different ways. I had matured as a person, grown as a woman and mother, and had tremendous growth in my own faith. Without those dreams and without the birth of both my daughters, I would never have ended up being the person I had become on that very day. I picked Faith up and touched every inch of her face with my eyes, looking at who she was, seeing my husband in her eyes as well as all her ancestors who manifested themselves within her too. What a magnificent thought that we humans are gifted with children. Each child receives our DNA and becomes a brand-new person. Each one of us is unique and knitted together in our mother's oceanic wombs, each hair counted on our heads. We are but stewards of our children; they do not belong to us. I had relinquished that power struggle to the Lord the evening before. We have only been entrusted to care for our children, to assist them in navigating the deep waters of the ocean they will one day be set adrift on when they become adults. It is our job to ensure they are outfitted with strong enough boats to get over the swells and through stormy seas so that they do not capsize and drown. For me, that alone has become one of the most significant and meaningful tasks in this world. I glanced out of the hospital window and up into the sky at the large, orange-pumpkin sun that hung lazily in the air. I searched for Him in the clouds that floated by hoping He would send me a sign of assurance that He had never left my side. Nothing. I looked and watched, watched and looked, nothing. Soon thereafter, Joey and Ruth joined us, and then our nurse brought Faith's discharge orders to us; we were ready to go home!

More than excited to leave, I gathered everything up, piled it helter-skelter on the cart they had provided us with, kissed both my girls, and sat down in the wheelchair with Faith on my lap and enjoyed the ride down the hallway and back into normalcy again. At the exit door, Joey took the girls from me and went to retrieve the car from the valet parking, leaving me to wait with our things there on the sidewalk, near the same place where Ruth had seen her Jesus sitting on the curb. I looked around anxiously, waiting for my crew to reappear, and spotted a lone chair next to one of the pillars near the valet's small, cramped cubicle space. Although there were many people waiting for their vehicles, no one sat in the chair. Its scrubbed metal frame and pumpkin-orange vinyl cushion called out to me like the sun in the sky, and I was more than willing to rest my weary bones on it. Coming closer, I saw that the vinyl seat was torn wide open on one side with stuffing thick as lamb's wool hanging out of it. Was this the pumpkin sun of my dreams split open to allow lava tears to drip out onto a passerby? The chair looked decrepit; it was a throw away, a chair with a defect that spilled its grief onto the pavement. A chair that no one wanted to sit in, but today, today that chair was beautiful to me. I sat down and enjoyed what the seat offered to me, comfort and a first-class seat in an arena unseen by human eyes.

As I sat waiting for our car, I took advantage of the fact that I had two children to look after and leaned back, closing my eyes. The trees began to rustle vigorously in a wind that mysteriously kicked up and swirled and danced around in the late spring heat. I opened my eyes and noted that the breeze was unusually cool and soothing with pockets of balmy warmth laced within it. It was a hot day out, and the breeze was so cool and nice, and it was then I knew that His angels were moving about on the wind. I closed my eyes tightly and smiled, enjoying the feeling of what I imagined to be silky robes brushing gently across my face. That day, I was not afraid to breathe in deeply. I was no longer afraid of hospitals and saw them as places of healing. I saw those angels in my mind, rushing back and forth, escorting souls into the heavens, hovering over the beds of the ill, guiding the surgeon's hands and supporting the weary doctors and teams of nurses in their daily routines. I felt them rush by with every balmy pocket of air and once again opened my eyes to watch the trees across the street applaud Him. I felt as if I was bearing witness to the trees' worship and awe as they unabashedly rocked and swayed to joyous music in a heavenly cathedral we cannot hear as the angels changed shifts at the hospital.

My beautiful pumpkin-orange chair had become a throne, the hospital, an altar. The chair was a perfect throne for those who could see it that way. The winds were His messengers, and the Trinity was a symbol of love to show me that He is always near. Now I got it! Through trials and many lessons in my life, I had come to learn what the gift of faith was by receiving the gift of Faith which unlocked the gates of grace in my life. I was going to be okay at this mother thing after all, and both my girls were going to be just fine. Their mother had been promoted to a full-fledged four-star admiral navigating her own battleship now, which traversed the rough seas with ease. Long gone was the leaky dinghy and sailboat with the unsure little girl bailing frantically. Now, in her place was a woman who had been given confidence through life's lessons, family, husband, children, and faith, to face and conquer more than she ever thought she could. I had learned the T*Ruth* about the gift of Faith from both of my daughters that I would always attempt to live by. *Mom, thank you for those words of wisdom,* I thought. *I followed them the best I could so that I could be the best at being a mother as I could. If there is nothing more in this world to achieve, I will be happy because I have truly been given a crown with two beautiful pearls in it.* At that moment, I could have sworn I felt her caress my face with her hand in the wind.

Knowing that about my new and much improved self, I got up out of the chair as Joey pulled into the circle, and I quickly looked up at the pumpkin sun that sat so beautifully in the sky. I mouthed the words, *"They found a uterus,"* and then laughed and said as loud as I could, "Thank you, God," as I ducked into the car to go home. It was then I realized that those two little sprites had taught me what true love really means.

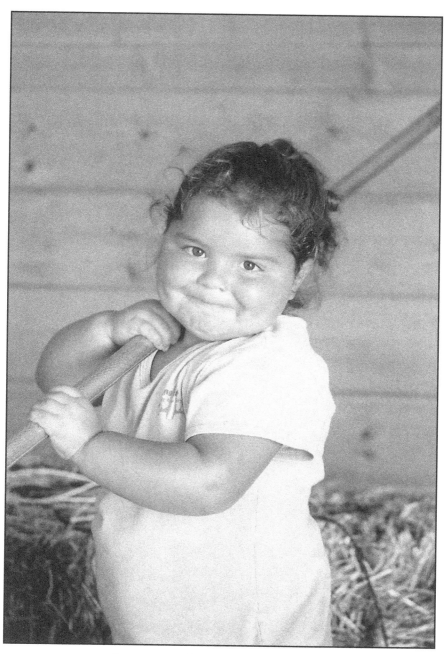

"I have something I want you to do."

~ God ~